THE COMMON COLD AND OTHER RESPIRATORY INFECTIONS • SORE THROAT • INDIGESTION AND HEARTBURN • DIARRHEA • CONSTIPATION • HEMORRHOIDS • ACNE AND OTHER SKIN PROBLEMS • BURNS AND SUNBURNS • POISON IVY (OAK AND SUMAC) • EYE PROBLEMS • HEADACHES • ARTHRITIS AND RHEUMATISM • NEURALGIA • MUSCLE ACHES AND PAINS • OVERWEIGHT • MENSTRUAL DISORDERS • INSOMNIA AND TENSION

This invaluable home medical guide tells you:

—**The symptoms identifying each of the above ailments, and the nature of each disorder.**

—**The effectiveness and possible side effects of the many different brand-name, over-the-counter drugs now on the market.**

—**The medications that are useless and even dangerous.**

—**The wide price differences for similar preparations.**

—**When you should consult your doctor.**

Written for the layman by an eminent physician, and arranged in easy-to-read tables for instant reference, this authoritative book cuts through all the competing, conflicting, misleading drug-company ads. It will help you protect both your health and your money.

A DOCTOR'S GUIDE TO NON-PRESCRIPTION DRUGS

MORTON K. RUBINSTEIN, M.D., a graduate of Harvard Medical School, is currently Associate Clinical Professor of Neurology at U.C.L.A.

SIGNET Books of Related Interest

☐ **THE NEW AMERICAN MEDICAL DICTIONARY AND HEALTH MANUAL by Robert E. Rothenberg, M.D., F.A.C.S.** This newly revised third edition includes a complete Medicare Handbook and up-to-date information on contraceptive drugs and devices in addition to over 8700 definitions of medical terms, diseases and disorders, a comprehensive health manual, charts and tables and much, much more. With over 300 illustrations.
(#E7055—$2.25)

☐ **EARLY DETECTION BREAST CANCER IS CURABLE by Philip Strax, M.D., Medical Director of The Guttman Breast Diagnostic Institute.** A well-known specialist tells you how you can protect yourself against the disease all women fear most. "Required reading for every woman."—American Cancer Society. (#Y6643—$1.25)

☐ **OH, MY ACHING BACK A Doctor's Guide to Your Back Pain and How to Control It by Leon Root, M.D., and Thomas Kiernan.** Introduction by James Nicholas, M.D., physician to the N.Y. Jets. Are backaches interfering with everything you do? Here is positive relief for you and tens of millions of Americans with back miseries. This wonderful, long-needed book tells you how you can free yourself of back problems—forever!
(#J6512—$1.95)

☐ **THE SILENT DISEASE: HYPERTENSION by Lawrence Galton,** with an introduction by Frank A. Finnerty Jr., M.D., Chief, Cardiovascular Research, D.C. General Hospital. Doctors who have researched the #1 cause of heart attack and stroke take you beyond **Type A Behavior and Your Heart** to show you how to save your life! (#E7200—$1.75)

THE NEW AMERICAN LIBRARY, INC.,
P.O. Box 999, Bergenfield, New Jersey 07621

Please send me the SIGNET BOOKS I have checked above. I am enclosing $_____(check or money order—no currency or C.O.D.'s). Please include the list price plus 35¢ a copy to cover handling and mailing costs. (Prices and numbers are subject to change without notice.)

Name_____

Address_____

City_____State_____Zip Code_____
Allow at least 4 weeks for delivery

A Doctor's Guide to Non-Prescription Drugs

By

Morton K. Rubinstein, M.D.

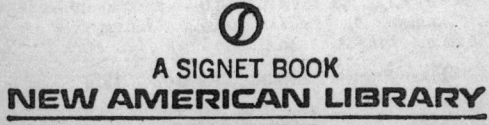

A SIGNET BOOK
NEW AMERICAN LIBRARY
TIMES MIRROR

NAL BOOKS ARE ALSO AVAILABLE AT DISCOUNTS IN BULK QUANTITY FOR INDUSTRIAL OR SALES-PROMOTIONAL USE. FOR DETAILS, WRITE TO PREMIUM MARKETING DIVISION, NEW AMERICAN LIBRARY, INC., 1301 AVENUE OF THE AMERICAS, NEW YORK, NEW YORK 10019.

COPYRIGHT © 1977 BY MORTON K. RUBINSTEIN, M.D.

All rights reserved

SIGNET TRADEMARK REG. U.S. PAT. OFF. AND FOREIGN COUNTRIES
REGISTERED TRADEMARK—MARCA REGISTRADA
HECHO EN CHICAGO, U.S.A.

SIGNET, SIGNET CLASSICS, MENTOR, PLUME and MERIDIAN BOOKS
are published by The New American Library, Inc.,
1301 Avenue of the Americas, New York, New York 10019.

FIRST SIGNET PRINTING, NOVEMBER, 1977

1 2 3 4 5 6 7 8 9

PRINTED IN THE UNITED STATES OF AMERICA

For my parents

Contents

Introduction x

1. The Common Cold and Other Upper Respiratory Infections 1
2. Sore Throat 17
3. Cough 23
4. Indigestion and Heartburn 35
5. Diarrhea 48
6. Constipation 56
7. Hemorrhoids 67
8. Acne and Other Skin Problems 76
9. Burns and Sunburn 89
10. Poison Ivy (Poison Oak and Poison Sumac) 98
11. Eye Problems 102
12. Headache 110
13. Arthritis and Rheumatism, Neuralgia, Neuritis, and Muscle Aches and Pains 124
14. Overweight Problems 139
15. Menstrual Disorders 151
16. Insomnia and Tension 161

INDEX 173

Introduction

The purpose of this book is to serve as an easy-to-use practical guide to the selection of non-prescription drugs (also referred to as over-the-counter, or "OTC" drugs).

Most persons attempt to self-treat their illness (other than emergency situations) for approximately two weeks before seeing a doctor. This is understandable since most symptoms resolve spontaneously with or without either medicine or medical advice, within a relatively short period of time. Further, the high cost of medical care precludes its use for minor conditions.

With thousands of OTC drugs crowding drugstore and supermarket shelves (more than 800 cough preparations alone), how is the consumer to choose the best product for his condition? It is obvious that any attempt to judge medicine on the basis of its chemical constituents will leave the average purchaser mystified. The vast majority of sales of OTC products are therefore based on mass-marketing techniques rather than on the quality and effectiveness of the drug.

In looking closely at the OTC drug market, certain features common to many of these products are apparent. In the first place, the effectiveness of many OTC preparations is strictly limited. This is so because the more potent medications are generally available only by prescription. Although there are exceptions, the OTC drug consumer should not delude himself into believing that he will be able to cure many of his problems with the use of non-prescription drugs. Generally, all he can hope for is to lessen some of his symptoms until such time as "nature takes its course," and the problem spontaneously resolves. This is not to underestimate the value of relieving annoying symptoms. When illness occurs, most of us are grateful for *any* relief we can get. It is this hope that makes the OTC drug market well over a billion-dollar-a-year industry in the United States alone.

Secondly, all medication carries certain hazards and it is

important that the treatment is not worse than the disease. This is especially true when minor problems, such as those usually treated by OTC drugs, are involved. The potential hazard of some OTC preparations is probably the best reason not to use these products indiscriminately. For instance, a large segment of the population is unaware of the fact that they have high blood pressure. Certain OTC medications for the common cold contain drugs which could raise blood pressure to dangerous levels in susceptible persons.

Thirdly, there are so many OTC products available for each condition (over 500 antacid preparations, over 800 cough preparations, over 100 "sleep-aids," etc.) that the consumer is led to believe (usually courtesy of TV advertising), that there are significant differences among the various products marketed for the same or similar condition. They may, of course, be packaged differently, i.e., sold in syrup rather than pill form, but the fact is that the vast majority of products for the same condition have little if any real difference.

The questions of effectiveness, potential dangers, and over-abundance of similar products are considered more fully in this book in relation to specific preparations.

It must be emphasized that no attempt has been made to list all OTC products. There are simply too many. Only the most popular ones are included. You may be surprised to see that many of these preparations are not as effective or as economical as some lesser-known ones. However, you may sometimes have a difficult time in finding the products you wish, or the ones recommended here. This is so because retailers carry the products which sell best, that is, are advertised most widely. In addition, there are significant regional and cultural differences in the purchase of OTC drugs which make it difficult to find a particular product in some parts of the country, or even in some areas of a city.

In this book, only preparations for the relief of symptoms are discussed. Cosmetics (including deodorants, mouth washes, etc.) are not considered. Do not be surprised, therefore, if a product you have been using is omitted. No implications are made regarding the effectiveness or potential hazards of any drug or preparation not specifically mentioned in this book.

The most economical way to buy OTC drugs is to choose brands that are sold either by generic (chemical) name or as "house brands." For instance, the cheapest aspirin available is sold under a variety of "house brand" names such as Safeway

Aspirin, Thrifty Aspirin, etc. These "cheapies" are generally every bit as good as the more expensive "brand names." Unfortunately, only the most popular medicines, such as aspirin, some antacids, etc. are sold in this manner, so that choice is all too often limited to the more expensive "brand names."

A Doctor's Guide to Non-Prescription Drugs is organized along the following lines: 1. There is an explanation of the causes of symptoms in each category. 2. The symptoms that are appropriately treated by OTC drugs are differentiated from those that should be brought to a physician's attention. 3. When self-treatment is appropriate, a specific treatment plan is suggested. 4. Recommended OTC medicines are described and are listed in charts according to their effectiveness and possible side effects. 5. When preparations contain unnecessary and/or ineffective ingredients, this is also indicated. 6. Finally, approximate retail prices for "recommended" and "acceptable" products are given.

These prices were derived from sampling Los Angeles' pharmacies and supermarkets, both large and small. They were then compared with the *1976 Red Book*, a handbook for the drug industry which lists manufacturers' suggested prices. An "average" was figured but, it must be emphasized, the retail prices listed here are only rough guidelines. They will vary from state to state, with store type and size, and with time. The major value of listing prices is to provide a cost comparison for medically equivalent products, so that when quality is similar, a choice may be made on the basis of cost.

Best use of this book is made by checking specific symptoms to be certain that self-treatment is a reasonable thing to do before seeing your doctor. Should you then choose to use OTC drugs, follow the suggested treatment plan and purchase "recommended" or "acceptable" drugs for your condition. Your choice should be made *before* going to the drugstore or supermarket, but carry this book with you and do not hesitate to use it while inspecting the OTC shelves. You will also find that most pharmacists are sincere and dedicated professionals, and can be quite helpful if you are having difficulty in choosing appropriate medication.

MORTON K. RUBINSTEIN, M.D.

Chapter 1

The Common Cold and Other Upper Respiratory Infections

One of the problems in discussing the common cold is defining it. Since all of us have experienced its miseries, we have some idea of the symptoms. However, the symptoms of the common cold overlap symptoms of other conditions involving the head, nasal passages, throat, and chest. In other words, not every running or stuffy nose, every sore throat or cough, is due to the common cold. It is important to differentiate the cause of these symptoms before self-treatment is begun, since the treatment can be quite different, and prescription medicine is sometimes necessary. For example, viruses are not sensitive to antibiotics, and so viral diseases such as flu and the common cold do not respond to antibiotic therapy. Strep throat, on the other hand, is caused by bacteria, which are usually quite sensitive to antibiotics. Thus, though the symptoms of these two conditions may be very similar, their treatment is quite different. Another example involves the use of antihistamines, which are very effective for symptoms caused by hay fever and other allergies, but ineffective for the very same symptoms caused by the common cold. This confusing situation can result in a potentially serious mistake in which a treatable condition, such as strep throat, is neglected, or in which colds are improperly treated with antibiotics. This inappropriate treatment can lead to serious consequences in some cases.

The major syndromes which are often confused with the common cold are outlined below.

Common Cold

OTHER NAMES: Head cold, upper respiratory infection (URI), cold
CAUSE: A combination of one or more VIRUSES

DURATION OF ILLNESS: 7-14 days
SYMPTOMS (not all symptoms need be present):

Most frequent

Nasal discharge
Nasal obstruction
Sore or dry throat
Malaise ("blah" feeling)
Postnasal drip
Headache
Cough (usually toward the end of the cold)
Hoarseness
Sneezing

Less frequent

Chilling and feeling of feverishness
Burning eyes
Muscle aches

Rarely present

Fever (if present, under 101° F. in adults, 102° F. in children)
Constitutional symptoms ("sick" feeling, vomiting, chest pains, diarrhea)

Flu

OTHER NAMES: Grippe
CAUSE: A combination of one or more VIRUSES
DURATION OF ILLNESS: 3-7 days (rarely up to 10 days)
SYMPTOMS (not all symptoms need be present):

Most frequent

Fever, usually over 101° F. in adults, 102° F. in children
Headache
Malaise ("blah" feeling)
Constitutional symptoms ("sick" feeling)
Loss of appetite
Cough
Muscle aches, including backache

Burning and redness of eyes

Less frequent

Sore throat
Hoarseness
Chest discomfort
Sneezing

Tonsillitis

OTHER NAMES: Strep throat, acute pharyngitis, viral pharyngitis, streptococcal pharyngitis
CAUSE: Either VIRUS or STREPTOCOCCAL BACTERIA
SYMPTOMS (not all symptoms need be present):

	VIRAL	STREP
Fever	Under 102° F. adults; may be higher in children	Usually over 102° F., both adults and children
Sore throat	Severe	Severe
Enlarged lymph glands in neck	Present	Present
Headache	Present	Present
Loss of appetite	Present	Present
Malaise	Present	Present
Pus on tonsils	Sometimes	Usually
Cough	Rarely	Occasionally
Nasal obstruction and discharge	Rarely	Occasionally
Earache	Rarely	Occasionally
Nausea and vomiting	Rarely	Occasionally in adults, frequently in children
DURATION OF SYMPTOMS:	7-10 days	Adults 3-5 days, children 5-10 days

Sinusitis

CAUSE: Bacterial infection of sinuses
SYMPTOMS:
- Pain and tenderness over sinuses in head and face
- Fever
- Headache (worse at night, better during day when sinuses can drain)

Allergic Rhinitis

OTHER NAMES: Hay fever, nasal allergies
CAUSE: Allergy to pollens in air (dust, plants, animal, etc.)
SYMPTOMS (not all symptoms need be present):

Most frequent
- Symptoms are seasonal, usually occurring in spring and fall
- Sneezing, especially in morning
- Running and/or stuffy nose
- Itching of eyes, nose and throat
- Redness of eyes and puffiness of eyelids
- Tearing of eyes
- Blockage of air passages

Less frequent
- Coughing and wheezing
- Asthma occurs more frequently in hay fever sufferers than in normals

The Cold—A National Expense and Nuisance

On an average, American adults have two or three colds each year and children, as all parents well know, are likely to have even more.

It is a fact that the common cold usually occurs in cold weather (thus its name), but the reason for this is not known. Perhaps it is because people are indoors and in closer quarters in winter and thus the virus can spread more easily. There is no scientific evidence that popular explanations for the development of colds such as chilling, wet feet, drafts, etc. play a significant role. Colds do occur in warm weather ("summer cold") but they are less frequent.

There are millions of colds in the United States every year (the incidence varies from country to country, for unknown reasons), and it is no surprise that there are hundreds of over-the-counter (OTC) preparations available for their treatment. Over $500 million is spent each year on OTC medications in an attempt to alleviate cold symptoms. There is no question that a cold is annoying and often debilitating. It is a major source of absenteeism from work—over $5 billion is lost each year in the United States because of this. In addition, there are untold numbers of ruined vacations and days lost at school. If we could spend $500 million a year on cold remedies and save $5 billion in lost wages and productivity, it wouldn't be a bad investment. Unfortunately, it hasn't worked that way; despite the money spent on treatment, $5 billion in wages is still lost.

Question: How much would be lost in wages and productivity if we did not buy any cold medication? Or if we bought twice as much?

Answer: The same—about $5 billion.

Is the Common Cold Curable?

The essential fact to keep in mind about the common cold is that, at this time, there is neither a cure nor a preventive for it. The cure depends on finding or developing an effective antiviral agent; the preventive will probably depend on proper immunization against those viruses causing the common cold. Massive doses of vitamin C have been advocated as a preventive and partial cure, but, as you will soon see, this is highly questionable. There is no doubt that it would be advantageous to be able to relieve the annoying symptoms of the common cold if it could be done effectively, safely, and cheaply. Unfortunately, at this time all that can be hoped for is incomplete relief of some of its symptoms.

Treatment of Colds

When taking any medication, it is important to keep in mind the seriousness of the disorder for which it is intended. The symptoms of the common cold have nuisance value, to be sure, and they certainly have economic consequences, but people do not die of colds and colds do not "turn into" pneumonia or other serious illnesses. (Pneumonia and colds can occur simultaneously, especially in the aged, but one does not cause the other.)

The common cold will last about a week if treated, and about seven days if it is not. At the most, symptoms should be gone by two weeks. We must keep in mind that we do not want to overtreat. We certainly do not want to use potentially dangerous medicines to treat a trivial disease. As in Gilbert and Sullivan's *Mikado*, ". . . let the punishment fit the crime."

The Pharmaceutical Industry's Solution

Manufacturers of OTC medicines seem to have a liking for combination preparations. That is, they put several drugs into each of their products, mainly to increase advertising potential and justify their cost. They would like to give us the impression that their single pill or capsule contains all the ingredients necessary to combat each and every symptom that you might now have or develop in the future.

This is contrary to the best medical approach to the treatment of disease. Physicians deplore the use of "shotgun" medicines. Generally, each symptom should be treated separately. It does not make much sense to buy a cold preparation that contains anti-cough medication if you do not have a cough, especially since the medicine will not prevent a cough's development. *All* medication can and does produce side effects in susceptible users, so the relevance of the ingredients is a prime consideration. Also, you may need more of one kind of medicine contained within a fixed preparation and less of another. It is therefore better to individualize the medicine, both in terms of specific ingredients for each specific symptom, and specific amounts for your particular case.

The Common Cold & Other Respiratory Infections

What Can We Do?

The table on page 2 indicates that major symptoms of the common cold are confined to the nose and throat. Malaise (that "blah" feeling) and headache may also be present. General aches and pains and muscle discomfort are more likely to be present with the flu than with a cold (see pages 2 and 3).

1. *Sore throat, headache, muscle discomfort, and general aches and pains.* By far the best OTC medication available for these symptoms is *plain aspirin*. Two or three aspirin tablets three or four times a day with meals or with a full glass of water should provide about as much relief as you will be able to find. Although aspirin offers more effective relief for flu (in which there is usually considerable body ache and fever), most people feel better on aspirin when "cold symptoms strike." There is one caution, however, to the use of aspirin for the common cold. There has recently been a suggestion that as little as two aspirin tablets, three times a day for five days, might lead to spreading of the cold virus to others with whom you come in contact. This is still a controversial and unproven issue. Whether or not you are more contagious, aspirin will very likely improve some of *your* symptoms.

2. *Nasal discharge, stuffiness, and postnasal drip.* These are the *major* symptoms of the common cold, and for these, over-the-counter medicine can provide significant relief. There are two ways to treat these symptoms. One is with local application of medication to the nasal passages by drops or spray. The second is with oral medication containing similar drugs. Medicines which act to shrink and dry the nasal passages are called "decongestants."

The most widely used decongestant is a drug called *phenylephrine*. When taken by mouth, *more* than 40 mg must be used by an adult to have any degree of effectiveness. In OTC oral drugs containing this preparation (Coricidin 'D,' CoTylenol, Dristan, Novahistine with APC, 4-Way Cold Tablets, and others), only about ⅛ to ¼ of the minimum effective dose is present in each tablet or capsule. This means you would have to take eight Dristan tablets, for instance, to get the *minimum effective dose* that could be expected to provide any significant relief from this over-the-counter preparation. However, because some people are quite susceptible to the side effects of this drug, there is a significant chance that nervousness, shaking, sweating, and dryness of mouth and throat might occur by taking so much medication. In large oral doses, the decongestants are likely to raise blood pressure and may be quite dangerous in patients with this condition (there are over 20 million Americans with high blood pressure, many of whom are unaware of their condition!). They can also be dangerous in patients with glaucoma or diabetes, and may also adversely affect patients with thyroid disease. Decongestants other than phenylephrine that are utilized in oral OTC cold medicines have essentially the same characteristics.

The local instillation of decongestants into the nasal cavities by drops or spray is generally safer but presents certain problems as well. There is no doubt that nasal sprays and drops such as Neo-Synephrine, Afrin, Contac Nasal Mist, Coricidin Nasal Mist, and others will temporarily relieve nasal congestion, dry the mucus, and allow for easier passage of air through the nose. Using drops or sprays also lessens the potential for systemic side effects, unless they are used in massive quantities.

The problem with drops or sprays, however, is that their action is quite short-lived and there is a great tendency to overuse the drug. All nose drops and sprays containing decongestants will produce a "rebound" of swollen tissue within the nose in a few days, depending on how often and how much is used. This invariably results in further stuffiness and blockage of the nasal passages, usually resulting in still more use of the decongestant in order to alleviate the worsening symptoms. Oxymetazoline and xylometazoline preparations (Afrin, Duration, Sinex-L.A.) are best tolerated in this regard, but they too, if used to excess, will produce "rebound" in a few days.

Drugs to Be Avoided

These are the two kinds of symptoms of the common cold—nasal problems and mild systemic symptoms—that respond to OTC medication. Judging by the kinds and quantity of OTC cold "remedies" available, simple aspirin and a decongestant are not sufficient, at least according to the "gospel" of the drug manufacturers. Almost all the cold preparations available also contain *antihistamines*, of varying quantities and types. This class of medicine can be very helpful in patients with allergies such as hay fever and asthma. The common cold is *not* an allergy. It is caused by a virus or combination of viruses. Antihistamines do nothing whatever to viruses, nor do they decrease the severity or duration of common cold symptoms. They may, however, and often do, have side effects such as dizziness and headache, and most important, can cause drowsiness, even in small doses. In fact, certain antihistamines require a prescription because of their sedative effect. The dangers at work and while driving are obvious, and *The Medicine Show*, a book by the editors of *Consumer Reports*, states that "antihistamines in cold capsules undoubtedly contribute to automobile accidents."

There are additional unnecessary components in many OTC cold remedies as well. Some preparations (Coricidin 'D,' Dristan, Novahistine with APC, Super Anahist, and others) contain aspirin and/or other painkillers, such as phenacetin (Super Anahist, Novahistine with APC, Sinutab, and others). There is some evidence that when phenacetin is taken over an extended period of time, kidney damage may result. We have already discussed the advisability of taking plain aspirin as needed, but these additional painkillers (there is no pain in association with the common cold) are not only unnecessary, but add a potential hazard.

Also contained in cold remedies are a variety of miscellaneous drugs, such as caffeine (for stimulation), antacids (for stomach upset), and others. None have any rational use in the treatment of the common cold.

Vitamin C

There has been a lot of hoopla in the past few years about the value of vitamin C (ascorbic acid) for the prevention and cure of the common cold. In 1970, Dr. Linus Pauling, a Nobel Prize winner in chemistry, strongly urged its use both for the prevention of colds and for reduction of cold symptoms.

He also claimed it would reduce the length of disability once symptoms had developed. Largely because of Dr. Pauling's influence and prestige, vitamin C has, in the past few years, become a popular form of self-medication for the common cold.

Since that time, there have been a number of studies attempting to corroborate this theory. Some studies have shown no effect, others have shown that the loss of time away from work or school was reduced with vitamin C intake. Many studies were inconclusive. One large study from the National Institute of Health (NIH) showed that "ascorbic acid (vitamin C) has at best only a minor influence on the duration and severity of colds..."

In 1975, scientists at the University of Chicago reviewed all the literature on the subject and concluded that "the unrestricted use of ascorbic acid [vitamin C] for these purposes [the prevention and treatment of the common cold] cannot be advocated on the basis of the evidence currently available."

Since Dr. Pauling recommends the use of over 300 times the recommended daily allowance set by the Food and Nutrition Board of the National Research Council, it is reasonable to inquire into possible side effects over prolonged periods of time. Dr. Pauling, and others, apparently believe it is safe, and that any excess of vitamin C is eliminated in the urine. The study quoted earlier from the NIH found no significant side effects. But in this study, only healthy subjects were used. Persons with diabetes or kidney stones and those taking other drugs or having other medical problems were excluded from the experiment.

Certain deleterious effects of vitamin C are known. For instance, it is well established that high doses of vitamin C can cause diarrhea. Also, since vitamin C increases the excretion of uric acid in the urine, susceptible patients, such as those with gout, may be more likely to form kidney stones. High doses of vitamin C may also change insulin requirements and thus be of great importance to diabetic patients. Large doses of vitamin C certainly produce false readings on the "testape," a common method by which diabetics judge their insulin requirements, or requirements for other anti-diabetic medication. High doses of vitamin C can also interfere with certain drugs and medicines, such as blood thinners (anticoagulants).

There is some evidence from animal experiments that large

doses of vitamin C may produce an increase in spontaneous abortions, and animal experiments have also suggested that vitamin C may wash calcium from the bones. Although not yet shown to be the case in humans, such calcium loss could adversely affect elderly patients with osteoarthritis.

In view of the fact that the common cold is essentially only a nuisance and not a serious disease, and that recovery almost always occurs within a week or so, it does not make sense to use high doses of vitamin C to try to prevent or ameliorate the symptoms. Its value is unproven; the possible side effects and dangers, particularly to the elderly and those with other medical problems, may be significant; and it is costly.

In view of these considerations, high doses of vitamin C cannot be recommended at this time for the prevention and/or treatment of the common cold.

Summary

1. The common cold is of nuisance value only, and does not lead to or "turn into" serious disease or have serious consequences.
2. At present, there is no known cure or preventive for the common cold.
3. OTC medication can help alleviate some of the symptoms of the common cold.
   A. *Decongestants* are useful for running or stuffy nose and postnasal drip.
   B. *Plain aspirin* are useful for general aches, headache, and malaise. (Aspirin, however, may contribute to the spreading of the cold to others.)
4. All combination remedies or preparations should be avoided.
5. There is insufficient evidence that vitamin C does much good, either in preventing colds or lessening the symptoms or length of disability once a cold has begun. The side effects and possible dangers of large doses of vitamin C may be significant in susceptible people. Vitamin C should not be used routinely for the common cold.

Suggested Treatment Plan for Symptoms of the Common Cold or Flu

1. Rest for 2-3 days.
2. Take plain aspirin, two tablets every 3-4 hours for general aches, pains, and headache. Be aware of the possibility that aspirin *may* influence the spreading of your cold to others. For those unable to use aspirin, Tylenol may be substituted.
3. For running or stuffy nose and postnasal drip:
    A. ADULTS AND OLDER CHILDREN: Afrin, Duration, Sine-Off Once-A-Day, or Sinex-L.A. spray or nose drops. Nose drops are used 2-4 drops in each nostril twice a day. This is most effective when instilled in nasal cavities while lying down, and remaining with the head to one side for a few minutes.
    Caution: Do not use Afrin, Duration, Sine-Off Once-A-Day, or Sinex-L.A. with: MAO inhibitors ("Nardil"), hypertension, heart disease, thyroid disease, or diabetes mellitus.
    Do not use for more than 3-4 days at a time.
    Do not use in children under six years of age.
    B. CHILDREN UNDER SIX YEARS OF AGE: Neo-Synephrine or Isophrin 1/8%, 2-3 drops in each nostril, three times a day. Head should be down and to the side of instillation for a few minutes. Do not use for more than 3-4 days at a time.
4. For sore throat, take plain aspirin as above, and gargles of warm salt water.
5. A steam inhaler or vaporizer using plain or distilled water may also help decrease stuffy nose and sore throat.

See Your Doctor If

1. Fever over 102°F.
2. Severe headache
3. Cough, especially if you are coughing up sputum or blood
4. Symptoms not significantly improved in a week

Decongestants

Note that "rebound" occurs when used for more than a week, and less in some persons.

GROUP I
Recommended Nasal Drops and Sprays

A. Adults. Dosage for drops: 2 to 4 drops in each nostril twice a day. Dosage for spray: 2 or 3 squeezes into each nostril twice a day.

Name	Form	Approximate Cost
Afrin	Drops	⅔ oz. for $2.53
	Spray	½ oz. for 2.28
Duration	Spray	½ oz. for 1.88
Sine-Off Once-A-Day	Spray	½ oz. for 1.59
Sinex-L.A.	Spray	½ oz. for 1.69*

B. Children. Dosage: 2 or 3 drops in each nostril, 3 times a day.

Name	Form	Approximate Cost
Isophrin Drops ⅙%	Drops	½ oz. for $1.60
Neo-Synephrine ⅛%	Drops	½ oz. for 1.29*

* Best buy in group.

GROUP II
Acceptable Nasal Drops and Sprays

Name	Form	Approximate Cost
Alconefrin	Drops	1 oz. for $1.53
Anti-B	Spray	⅔ oz. for 1.00
Clopane Hydrochloride Solution	Drops 1%	1 oz. for 1.70
Coryban-D	Spray ½%	½ oz. for 1.39
Gluco-Fedrin	Drops	1 oz. for 1.20
I-Sedrin Plain	Drops	1 oz. for 1.98
Isophrin	Drops ¼%, ½% Spray ¼%	1 oz. for 1.54
Mistol with Ephedrine	Drops	½ oz. for 1.35

Neo-Synephrine	Drops ½%	1 oz. for	1.59
	¼%	1 oz. for	1.39
	⅛%	½ oz. for	1.29
	Spray ½%	⅔ oz. for	1.79
NTZ	Spray ½%	⅔ oz. for	1.89
	Drops ½%	1 oz. for	1.59
Privine	Drops	1 oz. for	1.32
	Spray	⅔ oz. for	1.69
Sinutab	Spray	½ oz. for	1.39
Super Anahist Nasal Spray	Spray ¼%	½ oz. for	1.29
Vicks Inhaler	Inhaler		0.79

GROUP III
Not Acceptable Nasal Drops and Sprays

Examples of nasal drops and sprays *not* acceptable due to unnecessary and/or harmful ingredients. All contain antihistamines.

Allerest Nasal Spray
Contac Nasal Mist
Dristan Nasal Mist
Mistol Mist
Naso Mist
Soltice
Triaminicin
Va-Tro-Nol
Vicks Sinex
4-Way Nasal Spray

GROUP IV
Not Recommended for the Common Cold or Flu

A. Examples of oral combinations containing *antihistamines*

Alka-Seltzer Plus
Allerest Tablets
Allerest Time Capsules
Allergesic
Axon
Bayer Decongestant

The Common Cold & Other Respiratory Infections 15

Cenagesic
Chlor-Trimeton Decongestant
Colrex
Contac
Coricidin
Coricidin 'D'
Coricidin Demilets
Coricidin Medilets
Coryban-D
CoTylenol
Dristan
Dristan Time Capsules
Extendac
Flavihist
Midran Decongestant
Neo-Synephrine Compound
Novahistine Elixir, Fortis or Melet
Novahistine with APC
Quartets
Sinarest
Sine-Off
Sinustat
Sinutab
Super Anahist
Triaminic Syrup
Triaminicin Tablet

B. Examples of preparations containing *oral decongestants*. Be particularly careful if you are taking antidepressants. Do not use if you have high blood pressure, heart disease, thyroid disease, or diabetes mellitus.

Alka-Seltzer Plus Cold Medicine
Allerest Tablets and Children's Tablets
Allerest Time Capsules
Allergesic
A.R.M. (Allergy Relief Medicine)
Axon
Bayer Children's Cold Tablets
Bayer Decongestant Tablets
Bromo Quinine
Bromo Quinine Cold Tablets

C 3
Cenagesic
Colrex
Contac and Contac Jr.
Coricidin 'D'
Coricidin Demilets
CoTylenol
Covangesic
Demazin
Dristan Tablets, Time Capsules
Duadacin
Extendac
Fedrazil
Flavihist
Midran
Mistol
Neo-Synephrine Compound and Elixir
Novafed, Novafed A
Novahistine Elixir, Fortis and Melet
Novahistine with APC
Ornacol
Ornex
Quartets
Romilar
St. Joseph Children's Decongestant
St. Joseph Cold Tablets for Children
Sinarest
Sine-Off
Sinuseze
Sinustat
Sinutab and Sinutab II
Sucrets Cold Decongestant
Sudafed Syrup
Super Anahist
Triaminic Syrup and Tablets
Vasominic TD
Vicks Day Care
Vicks Nyquil Nighttime Colds Medicine
4-Way Cold Tablets

Chapter 2

Sore Throat

Like a cough, a sore throat is a symptom and not a disease. It is therefore important, before beginning self-treatment, to determine its cause. Sore throats can be mild, and are then usually described as a "tickle" or irritation, or then can be quite severe and interfere with swallowing, talking, and sometimes even breathing. They may or may not be associated with other symptoms such as cough, fever, etc.

Causes and Treatment of Sore Throat

1. *Dryness of the linings of the throat wall.* The linings of the throat (mucous membranes) are normally coated by a moist secretion (mucus). When these secretions are inadequate or become dried, the sensation of a mild sore throat develops. This drying condition is often the result of one of the following:
   A. *Decreased humidity.* This commonly occurs in overheated, dry rooms, particularly in the winter when the windows are closed. It is not uncommon to wake up in the morning with a mild dry or sore throat, for this reason. The "cure" is to keep the room a little cooler and possibly humidify it, either with a commercial device (vaporizer), or by using Grandma's technique of placing a pan of water near the source of heat.
   B. *Mouth breathing.* This occurs frequently in children, especially at night. Mouth breathing can be an indication of enlarged adenoids (glands at the back of the throat), but it can also be simply a habit. The constant passage of air over the throat (usually while sleeping) does not permit the mucus to stay moist. If a nasal breathing pattern is reestablished, the condition will clear up. Humidi-

fying the room will also help overcome this drying effect.

C. *Smoking.* Smoker's throat is caused by a combination of drying of the mucus at the back of the throat and the physical and chemical irritation of the smoke itself. Its relief is obvious.

2. *Infections*

A. *Viral infections.* These may be serious or trivial. A sore throat frequently accompanies the flu or common cold. You will know when it is due to an upper respiratory infection by the "company" it keeps. Colds and flu have associated symptoms such as fever, muscle aches, running and stuffy nose, cough, and hoarseness (see Chapter 1).

There is no medicine that will cure the sore throat caused by a viral infection, and relief, in this case, is completely dependent on the passing of the underlying viral illness. However, there are some things that can be done to make you more comfortable. The first step is to keep the throat moist. This is best done by gargling several times a day, or as often as required, with ½ teaspoon of table salt dissolved in an 8-ounce glass of warm water. Take a mouthful, throw your head back, and gargle. Repeat until all the warm salt water is used. Throat and mouth washes and gargles that are available without prescription are not any more effective than salt water. In addition, some can produce sensitivity reactions, and therefore, *none* are recommended.

A second way to provide moisture to the back of the throat is by sucking something that will melt slowly and thus coat the mucous membranes. By far the best and cheapest "medicine" for this is hard candy (*not* for diabetics), but cough drops will do. There are some problems with cough drops and throat lozenges, which make them less desirable. Some of these preparations contain antibiotics, and these should *never* be used. Antibiotics will have no effect whatsoever in eliminating a virus, but will increase your chances of developing sensitivity reactions to this type of "treatment." Furthermore, such cough drops and lozenges may make you less susceptible to the effects of certain antibiotics should you need them in the future for more serious infections.

Some states do not permit the sale of OTC cough

or cold remedies containing local antibiotics. California is one such state.

Another common ingredient of throat lozenges and cough drops is some type of anesthetic. Such compounds can produce a slight improvement in the discomfort of a sore throat, but their disadvantages outweigh their advantages. The four main disadvantages are: (a) that some persons are sensitive to the local anesthetic and sensitivity reactions are possible; (b) that they tend to make the entire mouth anesthetized, and most people find this disagreeable; (c) that their action is short-lived; and (d) that they are not very effective. Thus, cough drops or throat lozenges with either antibiotics or local anesthetics *cannot* be recommended.

About the only effective OTC medicine for sore throat is plain aspirin—two or three tablets three or four times a day with a full glass of water. It can be used in the same manner as it is used for treatment of headaches (see Chapter 12). Aspirin works by entering the blood stream and going to pain-controlling areas in the brain—yes, the brain, not the throat. Thus aspirin should never be rubbed on, coated, or used in any way other than by swallowing the medicine. It therefore makes no sense to use "topical" aspirin such as Aspergum.

B. *Bacterial infections.* One of the more serious causes of a sore throat is bacterial infection, particularly the type caused by streptococcus bacteria (strep throat). Sore throats caused by this bacteria must be diagnosed and treated properly because they can sometimes lead to heart disease (rheumatic fever), kidney disease, and other problems if left untreated. Unfortunately, it is not very easy to distinguish a sore throat caused by certain viruses (which do not lead to these serious problems) from a strep throat. A clue to this distinction is that sore throats due to streptococcus are *less* likely to be accompanied by the symptoms of a viral upper respiratory infection (e.g., cough, hoarseness, stuffy and running nose, and muscle aches and pains) and *more* likely to be accompanied by fever (over 101°F. in adults, 102°F. in children), fatigue, swollen neck glands, earache, and possibly rash. However, these are only clues and are not invariably true. Even experienced physicians cannot always distinguish between a strep throat and a less important viral sore throat simply by examining the patient.

The best way of diagnosing a strep throat is by means of a throat culture. A swab from the infected area is cultured in the laboratory to determine the type of bacteria causing the infection. A throat culture requires from one to three days for the laboratory testing, but does allow the doctor, with a good deal of reliability, to make the distinction between a strep throat and a viral sore throat. A strep throat can be effectively treated with penicillin or other antibiotics. A viral sore throat should not be treated with antibiotics.

C. *Other throat infections.* There are other causes of sore throats which may resemble strep throats or viral sore throats. Perhaps the most common one in young adults is infectious mononucleosis ("mono"). Certain yeasts (monilia) and the virus of herpes (cold sores) are less common causes of throat infections.

Summary

If the sore throat clearly is related to a flu or a common cold, it can be treated with aspirin, hard candies, and gargles. Waiting a few days to see what happens will do no harm. However, if a sore throat persists, and particularly if it is accompanied by fever (over 101° F.) or by symptoms such as earache, fatigue, rash, or swollen neck glands, or if it lasts more than a few days, you should consult your doctor.

Suggested Treatment Plan for Sore Throats

1. Associated with symptoms of common cold or flu (running or stuffy nose, muscle aches, fever under 101° F., dry cough, hoarseness):
   A. Plain aspirin, two or three tablets three or four times a day. Acetaminophen (Tylenol, etc.) may be substituted in same dosage.
   B. Gargle with ½ teaspoon of table salt dissolved in a glass of warm water several times a day, or more often if needed.
   C. Suck on hard candies, as needed (if you are *not* diabetic).

2. Due to dryness of throat caused by overheated room or mouth breathing:
   A. Correct the condition; humidify the room and decrease the temperature. Mouth breathing in children may be a habit or may be due to enlarged adenoids. Check with your doctor.
   B. Gargle (see 1B above).
   C. Suck hard candies.
3. Due to allergies or postnasal drip: See your doctor for treatment.
4. Due to bacterial infection (strep throat): If sore throat is accompanied by fever over 101° F., swollen neck glands, chills, earache, fatigue, or rash, or if it persists for more than three days without significant relief by using plan 1 above, see your doctor. *Note*: It is important to treat strep throat with antibiotics, since neglect can lead to serious heart or kidney disease.
5. Any sore throat lasting more than three or four days and not responding to plan 1 above: See your doctor.

OTC Medications for Sore Throat

GROUP I
Recommended

Plain aspirin

GROUP II
Acceptable

A. Examples of acceptable (but *not* recommended) throat lozenges or discs. All are of equal value. (Plain hard candies are preferred.)

Name	*Approximate Cost*
Cepacol	24 for $1.10
Chloraseptic	45 for 2.25
Listerine Throat Lozenges	24 for 1.25
Parke-Davis Throat Discs	60 for 0.69
Sucrets	24 for 1.29

B. Examples of acceptable (but *not* recommended) liquid oral preparations. (Salt-water gargles are preferred.)

Name	Approximate Cost
Betadine Mouthwash/Gargle	12 oz. for $3.84
Cepacol	14 oz. for 1.54
Chloraseptic	12 oz. for 2.25
Colgate 100	12 oz. for 1.42
Isodine Mouthwash/Gargle Concentrate	2 oz. for 1.95
Lavoris	14 oz. for 1.55
Listerine	14 oz. for 1.45
Micrin Plus	12 oz. for 1.54
Scope	12 oz. for 1.08
S.T. 37	12 oz. for 2.30

GROUP III
Not Recommended

Examples of "cough" drops or lozenges which contain local *anesthetics* and are therefore *not* recommended

Axon Throat Lozenges
Bio-Tetra
Cepacol Troches
Colrex Troches
Isodettes, junior, plain, super
Listerine Cough Control
Spec-T
Sucrets Cough Control
Trokettes

Chapter 3

Cough

Coughing is basically an explosive release of air from the lungs. It is generally caused by an irritation either of the linings of the air passages within the lungs, or of the lungs themselves. It can be either a voluntary activity or an involuntary reflex, depending on the severity of the irritation. Because coughing is an *indicator* of irritation within the lungs and air passages, and not a disease in itself, the cause of the irritation should *always* be determined.

The coughing mechanism is very useful and is nature's way of clearing our air passages so we can breathe more freely. This is especially necessary in life-endangering situations where food or foreign objects have become lodged in the windpipe. A similar function is served by coughing in conjunction with a cold or other upper respiratory infection where postnasal drip or mucous secretions cause irritation of the air passages. Some people cough from nervousness when in a situation of temporary stress, and some people, fortunately few, cough more or less continuously as a nervous habit.

Of utmost importance in any situation where cough exists is the fact that cough can be an indication or early symptom of serious disease. For instance, heavy smokers frequently are troubled with cough, and although "smoker's cough" may be the explanation, other causes *must* be considered as smokers (*especially* smokers) may develop other serious diseases—such as lung cancer—of which coughing can be the first symptom.

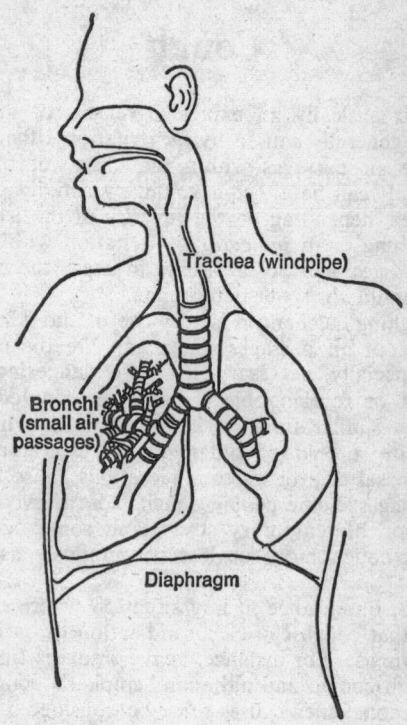

FIGURE 1
Respiratory System

Causes of Cough

Some of the causes of cough are:

1. Upper respiratory infections such as flu, and the end stages of the common cold
2. Bacterial or viral infections of the lungs or air passages such as pneumonia or bronchitis
3. Lung infections by tuberculosis or certain yeasts
4. Tumors of the lung or air passages
5. Blood clots in the lung
6. Irritation of lungs and air passages due to toxins such as cigarette smoke and certain chemicals; also job-related irritants such as coal dust, paint sprays, and other aerosols
7. Allergies
8. Heart disease and heart failure
9. Lung diseases such as emphysema
10. Nervousness

There are other causes as well, but the vast majority of coughs are related to one or more of these underlying conditions.

See your doctor promptly if any of the following occurs:

1. Blood is coughed up. It may be either red or rusty in color, and either mixed in the sputum or in clots.
2. Fever, weight loss, or shortness of breath is present.
3. Severe pain is experienced with the coughing.
4. Sputum is produced which is foul-smelling or -tasting.
5. There is a change in the pattern of your coughing.
6. The cough persists for more than ten days.
7. The cough is not suppressed by OTC preparations.
8. Fainting occurs in association with the cough.

OTC medication can be used to suppress coughs if they are caused by nonserious diseases, such as the common cold or flu. Masking or suppressing a cough caused by irritation of the air passages due to tumor or other serious disease can delay diagnosis and proper treatment.

Types of Cough and Their Significance

Cough is usually divided into two main categories: nonproductive ("dry"), or productive, in which sputum is raised. This distinction, however, does not necessarily indicate the cause of the problem. For example, a dry cough can accompany the late stages of the common cold and this same type of dry cough can also be present in the *early* stages of more serious diseases such as cancer of the lung, tuberculosis, etc. In determining the significance of the cough you should consider the context in which the cough occurs. If the symptoms of the common cold have been present for four or five days and a dry cough develops lasting another few days to a week, it is safe to assume that the cough is due to the cold and is therefore not serious. On the other hand, if a cough productive of foul-smelling and foul-tasting sputum develops in conjunction with fever, it is likely that the cough is due to bacterial infection of the lungs and/or air passages. Also consider any change in habit. If you are still a cigarette smoker and have had a dry "smoker's cough" for years, it is probably due to the irritation of the air passages by the cigarette smoke and its toxins. However, if the nature or the intensity of the cough pattern changes so that the cough becomes more frequent or productive of sputum, it is time to see your doctor (and stop smoking!).

Treating the Nonserious Cough

When you have satisfied yourself that your cough is due only to a minor illness such as the common cold or flu, you are ready for self-medication. Before contributing to your local pharmacist's well-being, however, you may wish to try to improve your own by some simple but often very effective means.

For mild coughs or throat "tickles," sucking hard candy is frequently all that is needed to produce significant relief. Cough drops or lozenges are very popular; Consumers Union reports that 43 billion cough drops were sold in this country in 1973. Most of these have a soothing effect and a pleasant taste. However, they have *no* advantage over hard candies and are considerably more expensive. In addition, the cough-drop manufacturers are fond of putting in two ingredients that should never be used for cough: antibiotics and local anesthetics. Antibiotics are not only ineffective in this form, but their use may decrease their efficiency if they are needed at a later date for a more serious disease. Local anesthetics may produce a mild improvement in the symptoms of a sore throat, if also present, but they do not stop the cough and their disadvantages (particularly the possibility of drug sensitization) far outweigh their questionable advantages.

Inhalation of water vapor is an excellent means of controlling cough and loosening thick sputum. Although many devices are sold that vaporize water for inhalation, a simple tea kettle is really sufficient. The commercial vaporizers are convenient for nighttime use. "Cool" vaporizers, which give off a fine mist of cool water, and steam vaporizers, which heat the water and release steam, are equally effective. Use only plain water in the device. Do not add any commercial products to the vaporized water such as Vicks VapoSteam. There is no proof that they do any good and they may be harmful in certain persons.

If these inexpensive "home remedies" do not provide sufficient relief for a simple cough, you are now in the market for OTC cough medicines.

What Is Cough Medicine?

There are only two types of ingredients that have any rational basis for inclusion in cough preparations: cough suppressants and expectorants. The former act to suppress the cough reflex (centered in the brain), and the latter help loosen thick and tenacious secretions within the air passages, thus enabling them to be coughed up more easily.

Cough Suppressants

Dextromethorphan is the cough suppressant most commonly employed in OTC cough preparations. It is good medicine. When used in proper dosages, it will suppress the cough reflex over an 8-12-hour period. This is particularly valuable for nighttime coughing. Dextromethorphan is also quite safe (if used in moderation), although in a few people it may cause drowsiness and/or nausea. These side effects are uncommon.

The effective cough-suppressant dose of dextromethorphan for adults is 15-30 mg three or four times a day.

Other cough suppressants employed in OTC cough preparations have no advantage over dextromethorphan, and most are not nearly as effective. Side effects may also be greater.

Expectorants

For dry, nonproductive coughs, the best means of liquefying the sputum is the inhalation of either steam or cool vaporized water. However, if it is inconvenient to bring a boiling tea kettle to the office, there are a multitude of cough preparations that contain chemical expectorants. Unfortunately, the vast majority of so-called expectorants in OTC preparations are ineffective in their ability to loosen and bring up sputum. This is sometimes due to the fact that the drug manufacturers are not very critical about the chemicals they use, and at other times the dosage of the drug is far below what is required for effective action.

The most widely used expectorant in OTC preparations is glyceryl guaiacolate. This drug has been reported to be effective in loosening up sputum when used in dosages of 300-600 mg three or four times a day. The popular cough remedies generally contain about 100 mg per dose, only a third to a sixth of the effective dose.

A wide variety of other chemicals purported to be expectorants are included in OTC medicines, but none has been shown to be of much benefit at the doses employed. The best that one can say about them is that when used only occasionally, they are generally harmless.

A Word About Sugar

Some OTC cough preparations contain a significant amount of sugar. Although it is not a necessary ingredient, for most people it cannot be classified as a harmful one. There is one exception. Diabetics should check cough-preparation labels and be very careful in their use of those with sugar. There are several sugar-free cough preparations that are designed especially for diabetics, and these are of course preferable.

What About Cough Pills or Tablets?

Although most cough suppressants are in syrup or liquid form, there is really no need for this. The medicine acts through absorption into the blood stream, and suppression of cough occurs by its action on the brain centers that control the cough reflex. Tablets or capsules, which also are swallowed and absorbed, are therefore just as effective as and probably more convenient than liquid preparations, especially for adults. They are also generally less expensive.

Expectorants work, when they do, in a different manner. After they are swallowed, they are excreted into the air passages, carrying water along with them, thus liquefying sputum. As with suppressants, there is no reason to take the expectorant in liquid form, although this does at least provide some water which may, at the doses usually employed in OTC preparations, be the only benefit of nonprescription expectorants.

Are OTC Cough Preparations Sensible?

A few OTC cough preparations contain an effective cough suppressant, and most are combined with an expectorant. The majority, however, show the typical "shotgun" approach of OTC drug manufacturers, i.e., the inclusion of unnecessary and/or ineffective ingredients. The tendency to combine medication for all possible symptoms in a single preparation is foolish and sometimes hazardous. It is much more effective, safer, and usually cheaper to take specific remedies for specific problems, rather than to try to put "everything" in a single preparation. Some of the *un*necessary components of many of the more than 800 available cough remedies are:

1. *Antihistamines.* Except for the infrequent case of cough due to allergy, antihistamines are of no value in suppressing cough. In fact, antihistamines usually act to thicken mucous secretions by their drying effect—just the opposite of what is needed to relieve coughs and get rid of the excess mucus. Antihistamines also possess the side effect of making the user sleepy. As has been pointed out in the chapter on cold remedies, many auto accidents, according to Consumers Union, have been attributed to this type of medication.

2. *Decongestants.* Decongestants act to remove water and thus dry up secretions. They are exactly the opposite of what is needed when you have a cough. In fact, the best treatment for a cough is to moisten and loosen the mucus in the air passages, as this will greatly enhance the ability to bring up the irritating material by coughing. Although many OTC preparations contain decongestants, fortunately, most of the products do not contain sufficient quantities to make much difference if taken in the recommended dosage. If taken in higher dosages, or in particularly susceptible persons, of whom there are many, they can cause anxiety, nervousness, increased heart rate, elevated blood pressure, and insomnia. Decongestants should not be taken orally if there is any indication of high blood pressure.

3. *Alcohol.* It has been suggested that several of the OTC cough preparations owe their popularity to this ingredient. Some preparations have as much alcohol as wine and a few are 50 proof (25% alcohol)! Rationale for its use is that it acts as a nervous-system depressant—and this is certainly true. However, if you want to drink, there are better ways to do it. Alcohol has no place whatsoever in cough medicines, and can be quite hazardous.

4. *Aspirin and other painkillers.* Aspirin does not have any beneficial effect on coughs. Many people with an upper respiratory infection find considerable relief with aspirin when there is accompanying sore throat or muscle aching. But if you only wish to suppress your cough, there is no need for aspirin. There is no sensible reason for including aspirin or other painkillers in cough preparations. Aspirin is not without its dangers (see Chapter 12). Use aspirin when you need it, but do not be forced into its use by buying cough medicine that contains painkillers.

Suggested Treatment Plan for Coughs

1. For "tickle" in the throat and "clearing" types of coughs, suck hard candies, cough drops, or lozenges. Do not use any commercial preparations that contain antibiotics or local anesthetics. Ask the druggist. Hard candies are just as effective, better-tasting, and cheaper (see Chapter 2).
2. For dry, nonproductive coughs:
    A. Humidification. Vaporized-water inhalations from a tea kettle or commercial vaporizer. Use plain water. Do not use any commercial products such as Vicks Vapo-Steam.
    B. Cough suppression. Use products containing dextromethorphan, no antihistamines or decongestants, and little alcohol.
    C. Expectorants. Most preparations containing dextromethorphan also contain expectorants, usually glyceryl guaiacolate. Their value is open to question, but they are harmless if not taken to excess.
3. For coughs productive of sputum:
    A. Humidification
    B. Cough-suppression medicine containing dextromethorphan.

If any of the symptoms listed on page 25 are present, or if there is a change in the pattern of a habitual cough, or if there is no simple explanation for your cough (such as the common cold or flu), you should consult your doctor. Do not continue to treat yourself with over-the-counter preparations.

OTC Cough Medicines

GROUP I
Recommended

These contain dextromethorphan, no antihistamines or decongestants, and little alcohol.

Name and Dosage	Approximate Cost
Cheracol D	
2 teaspoons, 3-4 times a day	4 oz. for $1.65
Queltuss Tablets	
1 tablet, 3-4 times a day	100 tablets for 7.00

Robitussin Cough Calmers
  2 teaspoons, 3-4 times a day   4 oz. for 1.90
Robitussin Cough Tablets
  1 tablet, 3-4 times a day   16 tablets for 1.23
Robitussin-DM
  1 tablespoon, 3-4 times a day   4 oz. for 1.90
Romilar Children's Cough Syrup
  Follow directions on package   3 oz. for 1.65
Silence Is Golden
  2 teaspoons, 3-4 times a day   3 oz. for 1.65
Sorbutuss
  2 teaspoons, 3-4 times a day   4 oz. for 2.98
St. Joseph Cough Syrup for Children
  Follow directions on package   2 oz. for 1.09
2G-DM
  1 teaspoon, 3-4 times a day   4 oz. for 1.85

GROUP II
Recommended Sugar-Free Cough Preparations

These are sugar-free and may therefore be used by diabetic patients.

Name and Dosage	*Approximate Cost*
Sorbutuss	
2 teaspoons, 3-4 times a day	4 oz. for $2.98
Toclonol Expectorant	
2 teaspoons, 3-4 times a day	3 oz. for 1.73

GROUP III
Not Recommended

A. Examples of cough preparations that contain *decongestants* and are therefore *not* recommended

    Bayer Children's Cough Syrup
    Chlor-Trimeton Expectorant
    Codimal DM
    Coldene Children's
    Colrex Syrup
    Conar, Conar Expectorant, and
      Conar-A Suspension
    Coricidin Cough Formula

Cough

Coryban-D
Dimacol
Dondril Anticough Tablets
Dorcol Pediatric Cough Syrup
Dristan Cough Formula
Histadyl EC
Histivite-D Cough Syrup
Naldetuss
Novahistine Expectorant and DH
NyQuil
Pertussin Plus Night-Time Cold Medicine
Robitussin-PE and Robitussin-CF
Romex
Romilar III, Romilar Capsules
Triaminic Expectorant
Triaminicol
Tussagesic Suspension and Tablets
Vicks Formula 44-D

B. Examples of cough preparations that contain large quantities of *alcohol* and are therefore *not* recommended

Arrestin (10% alcohol)
Coldene Cough Formula Adult (15% alcohol)
Cosadein (20% alcohol)
Creo-Terpin (25% alcohol) and
  Creo-Terpin Plus (25% alcohol)
Dristan Cough Formula (12% alcohol)
NyQuil (25% alcohol)
Penetro Cough and Cold Medicine (10% alcohol)
Pertussin 8 Hour Cough Formula (9.5% alcohol)
Pertussin Plus Night-Time Cold Medicine (25% alcohol)
Trind (15% alcohol) and Trind-DM (15% alcohol)
Vicks Formula 44 Cough Mixture (10% alcohol)
Vicks Formula 44-D Cough Mixture (10% alcohol)

C. Examples of cough preparations that contain *antihistamines* and are therefore *not* recommended

Axon Cough Medicine
Chlor-Trimeton Expectorant
Codimal DM

Coldene Children's and Adult
Colrex Syrup
Coricidin Cough Formula
Coryban-D
Dristan Cough Formula
Endotussin-C and Endotussin-NN
Histadyl EC
Histivite-D Cough Syrup
Novahistine Expectorant and DH
NyQuil
Penetro Cough and Cold Medicine
Pertussin Plus Night-Time Cold Medicine
Triaminic Expectorant
Triaminicol
Tussagesic Suspension and Tablets
Vicks Formula 44 Cough Mixture

D. Examples of cough preparations that contain *aspirin and/or other painkillers* and are therefore *not* recommended

Conar-A Suspension
Coryban-D
Naldetuss
NyQuil
Pertussin Plus Night-Time Cold Medicine
Romilar Capsules, Romilar CF
Supercitin Sugar-Free Cough Syrup
Trind, Trind-DM
Tussagesic Suspension, Tussagesic Tablets

Chapter 4

Indigestion and Heartburn

Like most of the other health problems discussed in this book, "Indigestion" or "stomach upset" is a symptom, not a disease. This means that an abnormal process within the body has resulted in the particular subjective experience which you find disagreeable, and naturally you wish to remedy the situation. Before attempting to alleviate the symptoms, however, it is important to determine which underlying condition is responsible for them. This will help define the seriousness of the problem and direct you to a rational approach to treatment. There are many causes for "indigestion"; some are trivial, and some very serious indeed. Distinguishing between serious and trivial is not only difficult for the average person, but also frequently difficult for physicians as well. There are some guidelines that can help you decide whether you may self-treat or whether you should seek professional help. In general, the more serious the condition, the less effective are OTC medications. Thus, self-treatment of serious diseases usually is not very effective. Unfortunately, inappropriate self-treatment may delay proper diagnosis of more serious conditions.

Some of the conditions which may cause "indigestion" or "stomach upset" are:

1. Overeating
2. Alcoholic beverages, smoking
3. Toxic reactions to the ingestion of chemicals (accidental poisoning)
4. Reactions to infected (e.g., spoiled) foods: food poisoning
5. Diseases of the esophagus (food pipe); reflux esophagitis and tumors
6. Diseases of the stomach; gastritis, hiatal hernia, stomach ulcer, stomach cancer

FIGURE 2
Digestive System

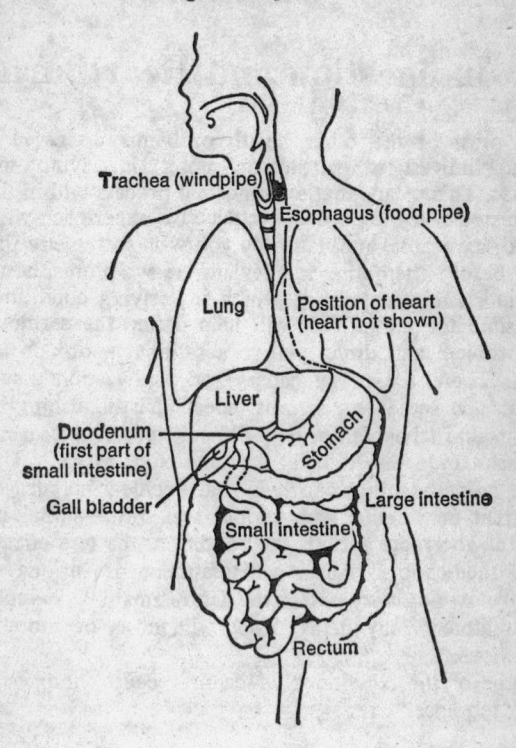

Indigestion and Heartburn

7. Diseases of the duodenum (first part of the intestine); duodenal (peptic) ulcer
8. Diseases of the large and small bowel; ulcerative colitis, diverticulitis and diverticulosis, regional enteritis
9. Diseases of the gall bladder; stones, infection
10. Diseases of the pancreas; infection, cancer, stones
11. Diseases of the heart (angina) may be confused with the symptoms of "indigestion" or "heartburn"
12. Nervousness

These are but some of the many conditions which may lead to "indigestion," "stomach upset," or pain in and around the abdomen. To be sure, most have special characteristics which help distinguish them, although some cannot be diagnosed properly without special tests and X-rays.

If *any* of the following occurs, see your doctor and do not try to treat yourself:

1. Vomiting for more than one or two days
2. Blood in the vomitus
3. Difficulty in swallowing
4. Severe pain in abdomen
5. Pain radiating either around the rib cage to the back, or straight through from front to back
6. Weight loss
7. Pain on manually pressing the abdomen
8. Abdominal pain relieved with ingestion of food
9. Abdominal pain brought on by eating, especially fatty foods
10. Unexplained diarrhea lasting more than a few days
11. Any blood in the stool
12. Large quantities of mucus in the stool

These are all symptoms of potentially serious disease for which medical advice should be sought. Your doctor may prescribe antacids for some of these, but he will do so in conjunction with other treatment and in a rational way.

Stomach Acidity

If you would believe TV commercials, we should have a national campaign for the reduction of stomach acidity. The fact is that large quantities of acid are essential for normal digestion. However, under certain conditions, stomach acid can produce problems. People with peptic (duodenal) ulcers are all "hypersecreters," i.e., they produce more than the normal amount of acid. This may lead to ulceration of the lining of the wall of the duodenum (which is the first part of the intestine, leading from the stomach), because this area is not naturally protected against high contents of acid, as is the stomach wall itself. Like the duodenal or peptic ulcer, the wall of the food pipe (esophagus) which leads into the stomach can be irritated if stomach acid acts on it, since it too does not have a natural acid-resistant lining. This is an extremely common cause of "heartburn" or "indigestion," and is termed reflux esophagitis.

The acid in the stomach, even in normal amounts, can cause pain if it acts on those areas of the stomach lining which have temporarily lost their protective coating, such as with inflammation of the stomach wall (gastritis). Some people have small defects in the muscle of the diaphragm near the junction of the esophagus and stomach, and the stomach can slip up into the area normally occupied by the esophagus, causing discomfort and irritation, especially when the victim lies flat. This is called hiatal hernia.

When Are Antacids Useful and Appropriate?

Stomach upset, indigestion, acid indigestion, acid stomach, stomachache, stomach distress, dyspepsia, and heartburn are some of the terms used in advertising media in attempts to sell antacids to the public. They are all rather ambiguous terms and it would be difficult to define any of them precisely. However, we all know from personal experience more or less what the manufacturers of antacids are trying to convey. They are suggesting that any deviation from normal, any sensations in and around the abdomen, can be relieved or lessened by taking antacids. The Federal Food and Drug Administration has forced these advertisers to use such terms as "temporary relief," "minor distress," etc., but these qualifiers are rarely taken very seriously by the consumer.

Antacids as an OTC product and home remedy can be very useful in certain conditions. When there is a sense of fullness or discomfort in the upper abdomen or under the breastbone that has resulted from a specific cause such as overeating or overdrinking, antacids may give considerable

Indigestion and Heartburn 39

relief until the process has had an opportunity to "settle down" by itself. When there is stomach upset or indigestion on a more chronic basis, such as with nervousness, gastritis, peptic ulcer, hiatal hernia, or reflux esophagitis, antacids will also be of value. If the symptom is recurrent (even though it is relieved by antacids), your doctor should diagnose the problem, since there may be additional steps he can recommend to effect a more permanent cure.

Of all the causes listed in the first section, antacids are most commonly helpful when used for indigestion caused by:

1. Overeating and overdrinking
2. Reflux esophagitis and hiatal hernia
3. Gastritis and peptic ulcer
4. "Nervous" stomach

Antacids used properly can help the symptoms of all these problems. But taking the advice of television commercials and using antacids at the first sign of discomfort has its dangers as well. For instance, stomach cancer sometimes begins as a gnawing, uncomfortable sensation in the abdomen. It is obvious that antacids will not cure cancer, but antacids may reduce the discomfort temporarily. This can result in some delay of proper diagnosis—a delay which may cost you your life. Likewise, certain forms of heart disease (angina) may appear to be "indigestion" to the victim; again, the use of antacids may only delay proper diagnosis. It cannot be sufficiently stressed that the cause of each symptom should be investigated before self-treatment is relied upon. The extreme would be to have a complete medical checkup with extensive laboratory and X-ray examinations for each little ache and pain. Obviously this is impractical, costly, and unnecessary. However, you do want to be reasonably certain that you do not have a serious disease before embarking on a program of self-treatment.

How Do Antacids Work?

Basically, antacids work by reducing acidity in the stomach. There may be other effects of antacids, such as coating the stomach wall, or reducing pepsin, another substance normally found in the stomach which may also have a part in the production of peptic ulcers. Antacids are thus appropriate therapy for those conditions in which symptoms are caused by excess acid acting on diseased areas of the stomach (gastritis) or an area where there is *normally* very little protection against acid (esophagus and duodenum). Antacids can reduce the degree of acidity and thus relieve the symptoms.

The ideal antacid is one that acts promptly, neutralizes a good deal of acid for its weight, lasts a long time, is not absorbed readily into the blood stream (thus avoiding systemic effects), has no side effects, and is cheap. The fact that so many preparations are on the market suggests that no single antacid meets all these requirements.

What Do Antacids Contain?

With over 500 commercial antacid preparations on the OTC market, which one should you choose? Antacid ingredients are usually in one of four basic forms: (1) magnesium, (2) aluminum, (3) sodium bicarbonate, or (4) calcium. The two ingredients that come closest to the ideal antacid (but do not completely meet the requirements) are magnesium hydroxide and aluminum hydroxide.

Magnesium and/or Aluminum

These two ingredients are usually marketed as magnesium hydroxide, magnesium carbonate, magnesium trisilicate, or aluminum hydroxide. Taken alone, the magnesium preparations such as milk of magnesia can act as a cathartic or laxative if used in sufficient quantities, or if used by susceptible people. In fact, Phillips' Milk of Magnesia is advertised as both an antacid (at lower dose) and as a laxative (at higher dose), and this is true. The aluminum (with calcium) preparations, on the other hand (Aludrox, Amphojel, Rolaids, Titralac liquid, Tums), are generally constipating. It was not long ago that two antacids, one containing magnesium and the other containing aluminum and/or calcium products, would be prescribed together. The patient was then expected to titrate or juggle the two in whatever proportion was most effective in producing normal bowel movements. The better OTC preparations now combine both magnesium and aluminum antacids in reasonable proportions, and these combined preparations appear to work quite well in most people.

Examples of combined magnesium and aluminum products are: Creamalin, Maalox, Magnesium-Aluminum Hydroxide Gel USP, Mylanta, and Mylanta-II.

Sodium Bicarbonate

Sodium bicarbonate has probably been used more than any other antacid as a home remedy for "upset stomach" and "indigestion." However, it is not a particularly good antacid. In the first place, its effects are very short-lived. More important, it can produce kidney stones and other difficulties if overused in conjunction with a large intake of milk (as many ulcer patients may do). It also has a high concentration of sodium, which is readily absorbed into the blood stream. This can be dangerous in persons with high blood pressure, heart disease, kidney disease, and other medical problems. It is best to avoid sodium bicarbonate in any form, either as plain baking soda or in OTC preparations such as Alka-Seltzer, Eno, and Fizrin. Rolaids are especially high in sodium, as are Phosphal-jel, BiSoDol powder, and Magnesium-Aluminum Hydroxide Gel USP. Di-Gel, Gelusil, Maalox, and Mylanta are all low in sodium. Tums and Pepto-Bismol tablets (Pepto-Bismol liquid is *not* an antacid) are two tablet forms that are also low in sodium.

Calcium

Such products as Tums and Pepto-Bismol tablets are calcium-containing products (usually as calcium carbonate). They have an intermediate value between the magnesium and aluminum preparations and the sodium bicarbonate products. They are constipating and are somewhat absorbed into the blood stream. Unlike most other types of antacids, they produce an acid "rebound." This is an increased acid concentration in the stomach several hours after ingestion. They are generally not the best antacids to use.

Other Ingredients

As usual, many OTC drug manufacturers contaminate their products with unnecessary and/or potentially harmful drugs. It seems obvious that aspirin should not be included in antacid preparations since aspirin can be irritating to the stomach (see Chapter 12). It can cause stomach bleeding if used to excess, and thus is especially dangerous for patients with peptic ulcers. Yet, Alka-Seltzer and Fizrin contain aspirin as well as an antacid!

Another example of irrational formulation is Bromo-Seltzer, which contains caffeine, which is known to increase stomach-acid secretion. Bromo-Seltzer contains sodium bicarbonate (a poor choice for an antacid), intended to reduce stomach acid, but at the same time contains an ingredient (caffeine) which acts to increase stomach acid. The logic in this is a bit puzzling, to say the least.

Simethicone is a relatively recent addition to some OTC antacid preparations. It is advertised to "relieve gas." It works, at least in the test tube, by breaking up small bubbles and forming larger ones from them. These large bubbles are said to be more easily expelled from the stomach than small ones. It is difficult to be certain whether simethicone is really effective for those conditions requiring antacids, but the product appears to be harmless and some patients believe it has some advantage over plain antacid. Di-Gel, Maalox Plus, and Mylanta are the three most popular products containing an effective antacid plus simethicone.

Proper Use of Antacids

Liquid preparations are to be preferred over tablets or powders. They work more quickly and probably last longer. There is also the possibility that a tablet can be passed out of the stomach before it has a chance to dissolve.

Food will neutralize stomach acid temporarily, but there is a rebound, or increase in acid, several hours after eating. Thus, the proper way to use antacids is to take an ounce of liquid preparation such as Mylanta one hour after eating, and then two hours after that. In other words, 1 ounce taken one

Indigestion and Heartburn

hour and then three hours after each meal with a double dose before retiring.

If you have any medical conditions such as high blood pressure, kidney disease, and so on, you should check with your doctor before taking *any* antacid. Although this is true of all systemic problems, it is particularly true of kidney diseases since even the most effective low-sodium antacids such as magnesium preparations contain sufficient magnesium to be detrimental to the kidney patient.

In any event, do not use antacids on a habitual basis. All of them can cause problems if used to excess, even in otherwise healthy people. If you feel the need for antacids for more than two weeks at a time, check with your doctor.

Additional Advice for People With Chronic Indigestion

1. See your doctor. Be certain it is nothing serious.
2. Do not try to alleviate indigestion by eating or by drinking milk. This might afford temporary relief, but *all* food produces a "rebound" of stomach acid, i.e., increased stomach acidity several hours after eating. Antacids are better neutralizers of acid than food.
3. Likewise, bedtime snacks will produce an increase in acid when you least appreciate it, i.e., several hours after you fall asleep. Take an extra dose of antacid before retiring if nighttime indigestion is a problem.
4. Caffeine in coffee, tea, and cola drinks stimulates stomach acid, and these are best avoided if you are troubled by indigestion.
5. Smoking probably increases stomach acidity as well, but to a lesser degree than caffeine.
6. Anxiety certainly affects stomach acidity, and should be controlled, if possible.

Suggested Treatment Plan

1. Check with the list of symptoms on page 37. If any are present, see your doctor.
2. If none of these symptoms are present, you may use:

A. Di-Gel liquid, Gelusil liquid, Maalox liquid, Mylanta liquid, 1 ounce (2 tablespoons) one and three hours after eating and 2 ounces before retiring.
B. Tablets are not as good as liquid. If liquid is inconvenient, tablets may be used. They should be chewed or sucked for full effect. Two or three tablets, one and three hours after eating, may be used. Di-Gel tablets, Gelusil tablets, Maalox tablets, and Mylanta tablets are best.
C. Refrain from coffee, tea, and cola drinks.
D. Avoid bedtime snacks.

3. Anxiety is important in the production of upset stomach. Try to control your anxiety or get help.
4. If symptoms persist for more than two weeks, see your doctor.

Antacids

GROUP I
Recommended

Examples of combination aluminum (and/or calcium) and magnesium preparations. Low to intermediate in sodium content. Liquid or suspension preparations are preferred to tablets.

Name	Form	Approximate Price		
Aludrox	Liquid	12 oz.	for	$2.16
Camalox	Liquid	12 oz.	for	2.40
	Tablet	50 tablets	for	1.70
Creamalin	Liquid	8 oz.	for	1.77
	Tablet	50 tablets	for	1.20
Delcid	Liquid	8 oz.	for	2.36
Di-Gel	Liquid†	12 oz.	for	2.19
	Tablet†	56 tablets	for	1.59
Ducon	Liquid	10 oz.	for	2.19
Gelumina	Tablet	100 tablets	for	1.25
Gelusil	Liquid	12 oz.	for	2.03
	Tablet	100 tablets	for	2.28
Gelusil M	Liquid	12 oz.	for	2.20
	Tablet	100 tablets	for	2.50
Kolantyl	Liquid	12 oz.	for	1.89
	Tablet	100 tablets	for	3.40
	Wafer	96 wafers	for	2.25

† Contains simethicone.

Indigestion and Heartburn

Maalox	Liquid	12 oz. for	2.12
Maalox No. 1	Tablet	100 tablets for	2.12
Maalox No. 2*	Tablet	100 tablets for	3.54
Maalox Plus	Liquid†	12 oz. for	2.15
	Tablet†	50 tablets for	1.47
Malcogel	Liquid	12 oz. for	2.03
Mylanta	Liquid†	12 oz. for	2.13
	Tablet†	100 tablets for	2.13
Mylanta II‡	Liquid†	12 oz. for	3.19
	Tablet†	60 tablets for	2.21
Silain-Gel	Liquid†	12 oz. for	2.03
	Tablet†	100 tablets for	2.03
Wingel	Liquid	12 oz. for	2.19
	Tablet	100 tablets for	2.39

* Twice the amount of antacid as in Maalox and Maalox No. 1.
† Contains simethicone.
‡ Twice the amount of antacid as in Mylanta.

GROUP II
Intermediate Value

Name	Form	Comment	Price
Alka-2	Tablet	Calcium carbonate—may be constipating	85 tablets for $1.53
Amphojel	Suspension	Aluminum hydroxide only—may be constipating	12 oz. for 2.39
Dicarbosil	Tablet (0.3 gm)	Mostly calcium carbonate—may be constipating	100 tablets for 1.86
	Tablet		144 tablets for 2.74
Pepto-Bismol	Tablet	Calcium carbonate only—may be constipating	60 tablets for 2.49
Phillips' Milk of Magnesia	Liquid	Magnesium only—may cause loose bowel movement	12 oz. for 1.39
	Tablet		100 tablets for 1.64
Squibb Milk of Magnesia	Liquid	Magnesium only—may cause loose bowel movement	12 oz. for 1.08
	Tablet		80 tablets for 1.08
Tums	Tablet	Mostly calcium carbonate—may be constipating	1 roll for 0.20
			100 tablets for 1.29

Indigestion and Heartburn

GROUP III
Not Recommended

Name	Form	Comment
Alka-Seltzer	Tablet	Contains sodium bicarbonate; contains aspirin
BiSoDol	Powder	Contains sodium bicarbonate
Bromo-Seltzer	Powder	Unnecessary ingredients
Calcium Carbonate and Soda	Tablet	Contains sodium bicarbonate
Citrocarbonate	Liquid	Contains sodium bicarbonate
Eno	Powder	Contains sodium bicarbonate
Fizrin	Powder	Contains sodium bicarbonate; contains aspirin
Gaviscon	Tablet	Contains sodium bicarbonate
Magnesium-Aluminum Hydroxide Gel USP	Suspension	High in sodium content
Pepto-Bismol	Liquid	*Not* an antacid
Phosphal-jel	Liquid	High in sodium content
Rolaids	Tablet	High in sodium content
Soda Mint	Tablet	Contains sodium bicarbonate
Titralac	Suspension Tablet	High in sodium content
Tricreamalate	Liquid	High in sodium content
Trisogel	Suspension Capsule	High in sodium content
Willard's Tablets	Tablet	Contains sodium bicarbonate

Chapter 5

Diarrhea

We have all had loose, frequent bowel movements at one time or another, so diarrhea is not unfamiliar to us. Like most other topics in this book, diarrhea is a symptom and not a disease. It may be caused by one or more of a large number of problems ranging from anxiety and nervousness to cancer. The important thing is to determine the cause of the diarrhea before treatment is begun.

The large bowel is at the "rear end" of the digestive tract; only the rectum is closer to the exterior of the body. The digestive tract is essentially a hollow tube beginning at the lips and mouth and ending at the rectum and anus. Food and water enter at one end and are processed, digested, and utilized during the passage from one end of the tube to the other. The foodstuffs successively go through mouth, esophagus (food pipe), stomach, small intestine, large intestine, and rectum. The solid waste products are then expelled through the rectum and anus. The fluid character of the food helps the passage and digestion of the material all along the digestive tract. When it finally reaches the large bowel, however, a major portion of the water present in the food is absorbed into the blood stream for eventual excretion through the kidneys. Diarrhea occurs when:

1. There is decreased absorption of water from food in the large bowel.
2. There is increased secretion of water into the large bowel, as can occur in certain disease states such as cholera.
3. There is excessive motility of the large bowel. Although absorption may be relatively normal in this instance, the increased speed of transit of food and waste through the large bowel does not allow sufficient time for adequate water absorption.

Diarrhea

FIGURE 3
Digestive System

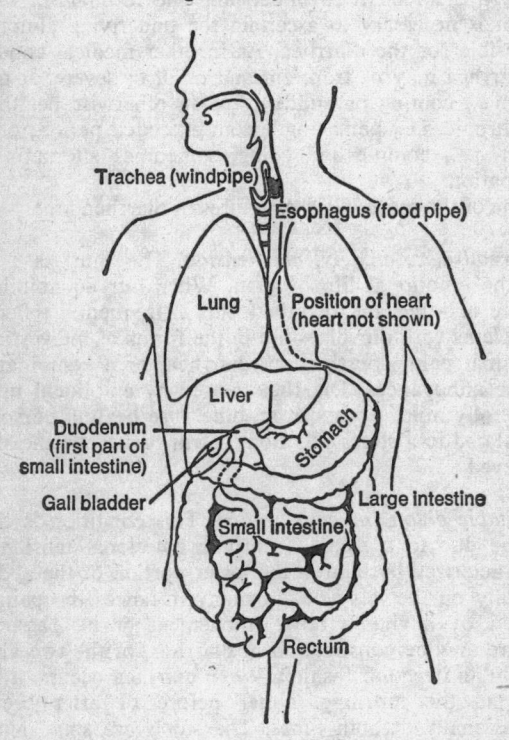

- Trachea (windpipe)
- Esophagus (food pipe)
- Lung
- Position of heart (heart not shown)
- Liver
- Duodenum (first part of small intestine)
- Gall bladder
- Stomach
- Large intestine
- Small intestine
- Rectum

Diarrhea is due to one (or more) of these three conditions. The basic mechanism of reduced water absorption from the large bowel can result in loose or watery bowel movements, or more frequent bowel movements, or a combination of these two.

It is not sufficient to understand the mechanism of diarrhea; it is necessary to ascertain the underlying abnormality responsible for the diarrhea. As in other medical conditions, the diarrhea may be transient and mild, or severe. It may be acute, i.e., coming on suddenly in an otherwise healthy person; chronic, i.e., persisting for an extended period; or intermittent, i.e., coming and going, sometimes alternating with constipation.

Some of the more common causes of diarrhea are:

1. *Nervousness, anxiety, and tension.* The "gut" is a mirror of the emotional life of man. When our equanimity and peace of mind are disturbed, this is frequently reflected in problems with our digestion in the forms of indigestion, abdominal pain, constipation, diarrhea, or a combination of these annoyances. Diarrhea caused by emotional upsets is generally mild, occurs in an otherwise healthy person, and is related to a stress situation. It will pass when the stress is relieved.

2. *Irritable colon (mucous colitis).* This condition is thought to be due to a state of chronic emotional tension. It is characterized by pain in the lower portion of the abdomen, usually on the left side. In many instances the pain is relieved by having a bowel movement or by passing gas. There may be constipation or diarrhea, or the two alternating in an irregular fashion. When diarrhea occurs, it is usually in the morning, either before or after breakfast, occasionally at both times. The stools are small and may contain mucus. In some cases mucus is passed without stool.

3. *Acute gastroenteritis ("stomach flu," viral gastroenteritis).* This, as the name implies, is caused by a virus or viruses. It occurs rather suddenly in an otherwise healthy person and is characterized by watery, frequent stools, sometimes accompanied by the explosive passage of gas. Abdominal pain is usually present, and vomiting is sometimes present. Fever is occasionally seen and malaise or a "blah" feeling

is almost always reported. This form of diarrhea runs its course in two or three days and then gradually subsides.

4. *"Food poisoning."* In the United States, this form of diarrhea most commonly occurs when we ingest food that "does not agree with us." It is rather nonspecific, but it is a common experience that mild bouts of diarrhea may occur when away from our own environment, for example, after eating in certain restaurants. Only very rarely does this occur after eating in our own homes. The diarrhea lasts only briefly and is of mild intensity. It may be accompanied by mild stomach cramps or other abdominal pains. It generally occurs within 24 hours after eating the suspected food, and if others who have partaken of the same meal also have diarrhea, you can be quite certain of its origin.

More serious is traveler's diarrhea, known by all sort of amusing names (Montezuma's revenge, etc.), but not so amusing if you are the "butt" of this joke. It has been thought to be caused by a change in water; the water may contain chemical constituents that our intestines are not accustomed to. However, it is just as likely to be due to an infection of the intestinal tract by germs such as salmonella or parasites such as amebae. This form of diarrhea usually does not begin for two to three days after ingestion if caused by salmonella, and for three to five days if caused by amebae. Fortunately, most traveler's diarrhea is self-limiting, though it may take several weeks for a return to normal. Some travelers, however, have persistent diarrhea, which, less commonly, is accompanied by a spread of the infection to other areas of the body, such as the liver. This can be a serious matter, and if diarrhea is not significantly improved in a week, a physician should be consulted, even when traveling in a foreign country.

Although this book is concerned with OTC medication, you should be aware of a medication that requires a prescription in the United States, but is easily available OTC in Mexico and some other foreign countries. This is Entero-Vioform, a very popular anti-diarrheal medication for travelers. It has been suggested that this preparation may be responsible for some cases of a peculiar eye and nerve disease, and in fact, its use has been restricted in Japan, Sweden, Australia, and the United States for this reason. Some of the names by which it is sold OTC in foreign countries are: Amebil, Bactol, Chinoform, Entero-Vioform, Enteroquinol, Iodo-Enterol, Mexaformo, Nioform, Romotin, and Vioform. When traveling, do not take *any* OTC medication for diarrhea that is not listed below.

5. *Drugs.* Certain drugs characteristically cause diarrhea in susceptible individuals. Antibiotics are particularly apt to do this, but so are other drugs such as magnesium-containing antacids and others. If even mild diarrhea occurs while taking drugs, notify the prescribing physician. Among other things, it may signify that the prescribed drug is not being properly absorbed, and thus is less effective than intended.

6. *Other causes of diarrhea.* The number of causes of diarrhea is in the hundreds. These causes include allergies to food (especially to milk), diabetes, inflammation, tumors, neurologic diseases, endocrine problems, narcotic withdrawal, and overuse of cathartics. As usual, it is important to determine the cause of diarrhea before depending on OTC medications for control of the symptoms.

If any of the following are present, do not self-treat; see your doctor.
1. Blood in stools
2. Black or tarry stools
3. Excessive mucus in stools
4. Severe abdominal pain with the diarrhea
5. Weight loss
6. Fever lasting more than two or three days
7. Persistent diarrhea
8. Intermittent diarrhea
9. Jaundice (yellowing of skin or eyes)
10. Any change in bowel habits for more than a few days

OTC Drugs Available for Treatment of Diarrhea

1. *Kaolin and pectin* (Kaopectate, Kalpec, Kao-Con, etc.). Kaolin is a gelling agent and helps produce formed stools. Pectin's mechanism of action in diarrhea is unknown. Kaolin and pectin are usually combined in a single

preparation. This is mild medication and will not be very effective if the diarrhea is severe. It is especially useful in children. Follow the instructions on the bottle for dosage. Adults usually require 2-4 tablespoons (½-1 ounce) after each loose bowel movement. Children will need less, usually 1-2 tablespoons, depending on the child's size. Do not use any medication for children under three years of age before checking with your doctor. Side effects: None in the usual dosage.

2. *Paregoric* (Parepectolin, Kaoparin with Paregoric, etc.). Paregoric is a mild narcotic preparation and is available in some (though not all) states without prescription.

   If plain kaolin plus pectin (Kaopectate, etc.) is ineffective, and paregoric is available OTC in your state, this may be tried for a few days before calling your physician. For adults, 1-2 tablespoons after each loose bowel movement is the recommended dose (when combined with Kaopectate), but should not exceed more than four doses per day without a doctor's advice. Children over three years of age can be given 1-2 *tea*spoons on the same schedule. Side effects: None in the usual dosage.

3. *Bulk-forming compounds* (Metamucil, Effersyllium, Mucilose, etc.). These are all psyllium-containing compounds which act to increase the bulk of the stool, reduce the watery quality of diarrhea, and thus make elimination easier. Psyllium is not too effective when used alone for diarrhea, but can be helpful when used in conjunction with other methods of treatment (see below). Side effects: None in the usual dosage.

Suggested Treatment Plan for Mild Diarrhea

1. Liquid diet. Avoid all solids, especially those with roughage such as raw fruits and vegetables. The exceptions to solid foods are rice and bananas, which may help to firm stools.

   Fluids should be the main intake during a period of diarrhea. These should be warm and salty. Fruit juice and tea are good. Avoid beverages that have a high sugar content such as cola drinks or sweetened tea.

   As diarrhea improves, add semisolid foods such as Jell-O, soup, etc. Do not return to a full solid diet too quickly.

In conjunction with a fluid diet use:
2. Kaopectate (or any preparation in Group I-A).
   Adults: 2-4 tablespoons after each loose bowel movement.
   Children: 1-2 tablespoons after each loose bowel movement.
   Children under three: No medication without doctor's advice.

If diarrhea continues for 48 hours, substitute:
3. Kaopectate plus paregoric (or any preparation in Group I-B). Use only if liquid diet and Kaopectate are not effective.
   Dose: Adults: 1-2 tablespoons after each loose bowel movement.
   Children: 1-2 *tea*spoons after each loose bowel movement.
   Children under three: No medication without doctor's advice.
4. If diarrhea is still persistent, you may try a combination of Amphojel (aluminum hydroxide), 1 ounce, four times a day, combined with a bulk-forming agent (Metamucil, or any preparation in Group 1-C), 1 teaspoon in a full glass of water, followed by a second glass of water, twice a day.

Drugs for Diarrhea

GROUP I
Recommended

A. Examples of kaolin plus pectin

Name	Approximate Cost
Kaolin-Pectin Suspension (various manufacturers, i.e. Moore, Pharmecon, etc.)	16 oz. for $1.50-2.00*
Kaopectate	8 oz. for 1.69
Kaopectolin	16 oz. for 2.03*
Pargel	10 oz. for 1.31
Pektamalt	16 oz. for 5.73

* Best buy(s) in group.

B. Examples of kaolin, pectin, and paregoric

Name	Approximate Cost
Kaolin-Pectin w/Paregoric	16 oz. for $2.52*
Kaoparin with Paregoric	4 oz. for 1.03
Parepectolin	8 oz. for 2.17
Kaopectolin w/Paregoric	16 oz. for 2.59*

C. Examples of bulk-forming compounds

Name	Form	Approximate Cost
Effersyllium	Instant Mixture	16 oz. for $5.30*
Metamucil	Powder	7 oz. for 2.42*
Mucilose	Flakes	16 oz. for 6.66
	Granules	14 oz. for 5.57
Plova	Powder	12 oz. for 3.75*
Syllamalt	Powder	10 oz. for 4.70

GROUP II
Not Recommended

These products contain unnecessary ingredients.

Donnagel and Donnagel-PG (Contain intestinal-tract "sedatives" which may cause side effects.)

Bisilad (Kaolin only, plus unnecessary ingredients)

Polymagma Plain (No kaolin, but does contain attapulgite—another gelling agent—and alumina gel. Not as much is known about this gelling agent as is known about kaolin.)

---

* Best buy(s) in group.

Chapter 6

Constipation

Constipation needs no introduction to Americans: TV never lets us forget it. No great service has been rendered the public in this regard. From a medical point of view there is almost never any need for routine laxatives or cathartics. This has not stopped the OTC drug manufacturers from marketing over 700 products designed to "keep you regular." They have been the cause of far more abuse than help.

It may come as a surprise to millions of Americans that bowel regularity is *not* a requirement for good health. There is a wide but normal variation in elimination habits. Many perfectly healthy persons defecate several times each day, while others—also perfectly healthy—may have a bowel movement only once or twice a week. Some persons are "regular," some are not. From a medical and health point of view, it makes no difference whatever.

Bowel movements are the body's way of eliminating waste products. Stool is formed in the lower portion of the digestive tract by the removal of water from the material in the large bowel. As feces are formed, movements of the large-bowel wall push them along to the rectum, where they are stored, awaiting evacuation. When there is sufficient stool present in the rectum, we feel the urge to defecate. This urge is highly variable because it depends on how much stool is awaiting elimination, how sensitive the individual is to the signal to defecate, what one is doing when he perceives the urge, how much and what kind of food and drink has recently been ingested, and, most important of all, what his lifelong bowel habit has been.

There is a natural tendency for eating to initiate the defecation reflex. Many persons have, since childhood, established a rhythm of elimination in which the desire to defecate occurs on a regular basis, frequently after breakfast. When this is the case, it is at least convenient; but although it is convenient to have a bowel movement on a regular basis, it is not necessary. However, when the urge to defecate is ignored because of occupation with other matters, the rhythm is frequently lost. The more the urge is ignored, the more likely it will be that the regularity of the urge will disappear. When the rectum is filled with stool, you will know it. Generally, when there is an absence of an urge to have a bowel movement, it is because there is insufficient stool ready to be eliminated. Trying to have a bowel movement when this is the case is like trying to squeeze more toothpaste from an empty tube. It is not worth the effort.

Constipation usually refers to the absence of a bowel movement over a prolonged period of time. There are certain situations when true constipation does occur. When there has been a long-established pattern of bowel movements and the pattern changes rather suddenly, it may indicate some underlying medical or psychological condition. For instance, certain endocrine, heart, neurological, and emotional problems are sometimes associated with changes in bowel habits. Also, tumors or cancer of the large bowel or other diseases of the digestive tract may change an established elimination pattern.

Common Causes of Constipation

Some of the more common causes of constipation are:

1. *"Irritable colon" syndrome.* This condition is characterized by intermittent bouts of constipation with the production of small, hard stools. Abdominal distress usually occurs and mucus may or may not be present in the bowel movement. This condition is thought to be due to long-term anxiety or other emotional distress. It may be due to preoccupation with elimination or faulty bowel habits, especially those established early in life. Treatment requires professional help, but it is certain that self-medication with laxatives and cathartics (which are a stronger form of laxative) will intensify and prolong the problem, and not prevent it.

2. *Laxative abuse.* There are a large number of people in the United States who feel that it is necessary for bowel movements to occur daily or every other day. There is no medical necessity that this be so, but these people begin to feel uncomfortable either physically or mentally because of infrequency (by their own definition) of elimination. Tele-

vision reinforces this notion, and a laxative is used. Many of the OTC preparations are quite effective and, indeed, a bowel movement is induced. In fact, it is likely that the bowel will pass more than the usual amount of stool with the use of these medications. The additional volume is obtained from higher up in the colon (large bowel) than where stool is normally stored. Thus, emptying can be quite complete. It will therefore take some time to reaccumulate sufficient stool to have the urge to defecate once more. However, this rather long wait for another urge to defecate makes the laxative user nervous and he again uses artificial means to induce a bowel movement. The cycle of laxative (or enema), followed by repeated laxatives, frequently results in destruction of the normal defecation reflexes with the accompanying urge to eliminate. This will, of course, cause further use of laxatives.

It is a terribly vicious cycle and although its cure is simple, it usually requires professional medical advice. The most important thing to do to break the laxative habit is to stop using them. A normal bowel movement will eventually occur (what else is going to happen to the stored-up stool?), but it is going to take some time because: (a) the bowel is probably well emptied out, (b) the production of stool does not occur instantly, and (c) you may have interfered with the normal bowel reflexes by overuse of laxatives.

You can help the process get back to normal by eating bulk-forming foods. Bran, as in any of the numerous bran cereals, is best. Just don't worry. A bowel movement will come eventually; it has to. When you do feel the urge to defecate, don't neglect it. Go to the toilet, if at all possible, but do not strain. Read a magazine. If the bowel movement does not come within ten minutes, forget it for this time and wait for the next urge.

3. *Constipation of travel and change of diet.* These are real phenomena but there is little reason to try and treat them. Such constipation will correct itself. Be glad you don't have diarrhea.

4. *Medical conditions.* There are certain physical and mental conditions which can lead to constipation. These include endocrine abnormalities such as underactive thyroid, neurologic conditions such as Parkinsonism and strokes, congestive heart failure, and tumors of the large bowel. Drugs such as sedatives, antacids, tranquilizers, and those used

for high blood pressure and for certain psychological conditions such as depression may also cause constipation.

Drugs that commonly cause constipation:

1. Codeine
2. Percodan
3. Pro-Banthine
4. Tofranil
5. Thorazine
6. Ansolysen
7. Inversine

When constipation is caused by medical conditions or drugs, the striking factor is a *change* in bowel habit. Should this occur, see your physician and let him be certain that the development of constipation is not a reflection of some underlying medical or psychological condition.

When Are Laxatives Advisable?

It has been emphasized that constipation is not usually a serious problem, and that it generally does not require laxatives, enemas, or cathartics. There are certain instances, however, when your physician will advise the use of laxatives or cathartics:

1. Before certain X-ray tests such as gallbladder X-rays, GI study, barium enema, or IVP (kidney X-rays)
2. When straining during elimination might be detrimental to certain medical conditions such as hernia, hemorrhoids and other rectal and anal conditions, heart disease, and others. If this applies to you, your doctor will recommend a program to keep your stools soft. It will generally include a diet high in fiber and bulk (bran, celery, fruits, and vegetables), and perhaps a laxative such as milk of magnesia.

If any of the following are present, do not self-treat—see your doctor:
1. Distinct change in bowel habits
2. Blood or tarry material in stools
3. Excessive mucus in stools

4. Abdominal pain
5. Weight loss
6. Intermittent diarrhea and constipation

Caution: Never use laxatives, cathartics, or enemas if abdominal pain is present.

Use of OTC Laxatives

Most of the OTC preparations sold for constipation do their job more or less effectively. The choice of which to buy depends on whether you need them in the first place, and if so, which one of the more than 700 products available will be most appropriate.

In general, you should do simple things first, such as a change in diet, and then, if necessary, resort to medicines. Should medicine be required, use the mildest and least harmful laxatives first. For difficult problems, you can progress to more potent preparations. Always keep in mind that the stronger the medicine, the greater the potential for harmful side effects. Since so many brand products are similar, price often makes the difference in choice.

Types of OTC Drugs Available for Treatment of Constipation

1. *Stool softeners.* These work by keeping the stool soft. They are best used when straining at stool is to be avoided, as in persons with hemorrhoids, heart disease, etc.
   A. Colace, Doxinate. Dose: two capsules a day. Side effects: none.
   B. Surfak. Dose: two capsules a day. Side effects: occasional cramping pain.
   C. Mineral oil (liquid petrolatum)—*not recommended.* Dose: 1 ounce before retiring. Side effects: absorption of certain vitamins; possible lipid (fatty) pneumonia; leakage from rectum (even when taken orally).

2. *Bulk-forming laxatives.* This type of compound works by absorbing water, swelling up and mixing with stool. They therefore act to keep the stool soft and relatively large in

size. The resulting bulk acts to stimulate the bowel to evacuate the mass. They usually work in 12 to 24 hours, although in some people they may take as long as two to three days to have full effect.

A. Natural:
1) Bran—bran cereals of all types (Kellogg's All Bran, Kellogg's Bran Buds, Post 40% Bran Flakes, Post Raisin Bran). Bran may also be purchased over the counter in drugstores. Bran should not be used by persons who have difficulty swallowing, since bran will swell up by the absorption of water wherever it is, and thus may enhance swallowing difficulty.
2) Bulk is also increased by eating foods with roughage (material that is not easily digested, but rather passed through the bowel more or less intact): celery, fruits, vegetables, prunes.

B. Synthetics: Metamucil, Konsyl, Effersyllium, Regulin, Serutan, Hydrocil, Mucilose. Dose: Take as directed with at least one glass of water, preferable two. Side effects: none.

3. *Salts.* This type of cathartic (stronger than a laxative) works by retaining water in the digestive tract. In the usual dose, salts work in three to six hours. They are used when milder laxatives are not effective and generally are best prescribed by doctors, although they are available OTC.

A. Epsom salts. Dose: 10-15 gm.
B. Milk of magnesia (Haley's M-O, Milk of Magnesia USP, Phillips' Milk of Magnesia). Dose: ½ ounce at bedtime. (Do not use either Epsom salts or milk of magnesia if kidney disease is present.)
C. Sodium phosphate (Sal Hepatica). Dose: 4-8 gm. (Do not use if on a low-sodium diet or have heart disease.)

4. *Contact cathartics.* This class of compounds works, at least in part, by stimulating the wall of the bowel, causing more rapid elimination of feces. They work relatively rapidly, usually in less than six hours and, depending on the dose, sometimes *much* less.

A. Castor oil (Neoloid, G-W Emulsoil). This is strong medicine and should be used only on the advice of your doctor, usually in preparation for X-ray procedures or surgery.
B. Phenolphthalein (Agoral, Ex-Lax, Feen-A-Mint, Pheno-

lax). Acts in six to eight hours. Dose: 100-200 mg. Side effects: may turn urine pink or red; occasional allergic reactions.

C. Dulcolax. Dose: 10-15 mg tablet (works in six to eight hours); suppository (acts in 15 to 60 minutes). Side effects: orally, none; rectal suppository, occasional burning sensation of the rectum.

D. Senna, cascara, and danthron (Doxan, Dr. Caldwell's Senna Laxative, Gentlax, Modane, Nature's Remedy, Senokot). These are thought to work by increasing intestinal motility, thus decreasing passage time of the stool. They take 6 to 24 hours for full effect.

5. *Enemas and suppositories.* These are generally unnecessary for routine, mild constipation problems. Although it might seem reasonable to place the medication right where it is needed, there are certain disadvantages to it when used chronically. Suppositories, for instance, can be irritating to the anus and rectal lining. Enemas, if used more than occasionally, can cause loss of reflex of normal bowel urges. Both can be habit-forming in the sense that a bowel movement will be difficult without them. On the other hand, an occasional enema or suppository is safe and effective.

A. Dulcolax suppository. One suppository will work in 15 to 60 minutes. Side effects: possible anal and rectal irritation.

B. Glycerin suppositories.

C. Tapwater enema is effective and harmless if used only occasionally.

D. Clyserol, Fleet, and Travad are conveniently packaged salt enemas. They may be irritating to persons with disease of the colon and have little to offer over tapwater enemas. They are also quite expensive.

E. Oil-retention enemas (Clyserol Oil Retention, Fleet Enema Oil Retention) are used for severe cases of stool-impacted constipation and are not recommended for general home use.

Suggested Treatment for Constipation

1. If there is a change in bowel habit, either to constipation, diarrhea, or a combination of the two, see your doctor.

Constipation

2. *Chronic constipation.*
   A. If you have been taking or using laxatives, suppositories, or enemas regularly, stop their use.
   B. Go on a high-bulk diet: fruits and vegetables, bran cereal (Kellogg's All-Bran and Bran Buds, Post 40% Bran Flakes, Raisin Bran, or other natural bran cereals), prune juice, celery. CAUTION: *Do not use bran if there is difficulty swallowing.*
   C. Do not neglect the urge to defecate. Try to have a bowel movement the same time daily or every other day. Right after a breakfast of bran cereal, prunes, etc. is best.
   D. Bulk-forming laxatives are mild and can be taken in conjunction with high-bulk diet. Metamucil, Konsyl, Effersyllium, Regulin, Serutan, Hydrocil, Mucilose are all the same. Take as directed with one or two glasses of water.
   E. If this does not work in a few days and you are uncomfortable, use milk of magnesia (Phillips' Milk of Magnesia, Milk of Magnesia USP), 2 tablespoons before retiring for adults, 1 tablespoon for children over six. This may be repeated for two to three nights in a row, if necessary. Sal Hepatica, Phospho-Soda, and Clyserol may also be taken as directed on the package. *Caution:* Milk of magnesia is not to be used in persons with kidney disease; Sal Hepatica, Phospho-Soda, and Clyserol are not to be used in persons on low-sodium diet or with heart disease.
   F. If you get no results from E, try tapwater or Fleet Enema.
   G. If no results from F, see your doctor.
   H. When bowel movement occurs, discontinue cathartics, laxatives, suppositories, or enemas *and wait.* Since you have now been cleared out, it will take several days for feces to reaccumulate in sufficient quantity to produce the urge to defecate. When the urge occurs, heed it if at all possible.

   Continue high-residue diet and bran. To ensure soft stools, continue to take bulk-forming agents (Metamucil, etc.).

3. CAUTION: *Never take laxatives, cathartics, enemas, or suppositories if there is any abdominal pain. Check with your doctor.* Children under six should not be given any laxatives, cathartics, enemas, or suppositories without an

OK from physician. Pregnant women should take no laxatives without a doctor's advice. *Do not take any laxatives, cathartics, enemas, or suppositories on a chronic or daily basis!*

Laxatives and Cathartics

GROUP I
Mild Preparations

A. Examples of bulk-forming preparations

Name	Form	Approximate Cost		
Effersyllium	Powder	9 oz.	for	$3.63
Hydrocil	Powder	4 oz.	for	1.90
Metamucil	Powder	7 oz.	for	2.43*
Mucilose	Flakes	16 oz.	for	6.66
	Granules	14 oz.	for	5.57
Plova	Powder	12 oz.	for	3.75*
Regulin	Powder	12 oz.	for	4.20
Serutan	Powder	7 oz.	for	2.24
	Granules	7 oz.	for	2.24
Syllamalt	Powder	10 oz.	for	3.36*

B. Examples of stool softeners

Name	Form	Approximate Cost	
Colace	Capsule	60 capsules	for $7.00
	Syrup	8 oz.	for 18.00
Coloctyl	Capsule	100 capsules	for 3.50
Correctol	Tablet (combined with stimulant)	60 tablets	for 2.49
		90 tablets	for 3.59
Dialose	Capsule (combined with bulk forming agent)	100 capsules	for 6.16
Diocte (DSS)	Dioctyl Sodium Sulfosuccinate (various manufacturers—Purepak, Spencer-Mead, Winsale, etc.)	100 capsules	for 2.10*
Dio Medicone	Tablet	50 tablets	for $2.49

* Best buy(s) in group.

Disonate	Capsule	100 capsules for	2.80
	Liquid	1 pint for	13.72
	Syrup	1 pint for	3.50
Doxinate	Capsule, 60 mg	100 capsules for	5.81
Regutol	Tablet	90 tablets for	4.19
Surfak	Capsule, 50 mg	100 capsules for	6.23

GROUP II
Intermediate-Strength Preparations

A. Examples of salts

Name	Form	Approximate Cost
Fleet	Liquid	6 oz. for $ .97*
Phillips' Milk of	Liquid	12 oz. for 1.39
Magnesia	Tablet	100 tablets for 1.64
Phospho-Soda	Liquid	6 oz. for 1.05
Sal Hepatica	Granules	7 oz. for 1.35
Squibb Milk of	Liquid	8 oz. for 1.13
Magnesia	Tablet	80 tablets for 1.13

B. Examples of contact cathartics

Name	Form	Approximate Cost
Calotabs	Tablet	10 oz. for $ .89
Carter's Little Pills	Pill	85 pills for 1.39
Dr. Caldwell's Senna Laxative	Liquid	12 oz. for 2.25
Dulcolax	Tablet	100 tablets for 8.43
Espotabs	Tablet	85 tablets for 1.49
Ex-Lax	Pill, chocolate	48 pills for 2.29
Feen-A-Mint	Chewable tablet	60 tablets for 2.39
Fletcher's Castoria	Liquid	5 oz. for 1.24
Modane	Tablet	30 tablets for 3.54
Nature's Remedy	Tablet	100 tablets for 1.49
Phenolax	Wafer	100 wafers for 1.29*
Senokot	Granules	8 oz. for 6.05
	Syrup	8 oz. for 4.98
	Tablet	100 tablets for 4.68

* Best buy(s) in group.

GROUP III
Suppositories and Enemas for Self-Treatment

Name	Form	Approximate Cost
Clyserol	Salt enema	4 oz. for $ .59
Dulcolax	Suppository	#4 for 2.17
Fleet Enema	Salt enema	2¼ oz. for .59
Glycerin suppositories (various manufacturers— DePree, Lannett, Winsale, etc.)		#12 for .60-.70*
Senokot	Suppository	#6 for 2.69
Travad	Salt enema	4½ oz. for .70
Tuck's Saf-Tip	Phosphate enema	4½ oz. for .60
Vacuetts	Suppository	#12 for 6.65

GROUP IV
Not Recommended for Self-Treatment

Name	Comment
Agoral	Mineral oil
Clyserol Oil Retention Enema	Mineral oil
Fleet Enema Oil Retention Enema	Mineral oil
G-W Emulsoil	Castor oil
Haley's M-O	Mineral oil
Kondremul	Mineral oil
Milkinol	Mineral oil
Milk of Magnesia— Mineral Oil Emulsion	Mineral oil
Neoloid	Castor oil
Neo-Cultol	Mineral oil
Nujol	Mineral oil
Petrogalar	Mineral oil
Petro-Syllium No. 1 & No. 2	Mineral oil

---

* Best buy in group.

Chapter 7

Hemorrhoids

What are they, what causes them?

The majority of adults over the age of 30 have hemorrhoids, and men and women are about equally affected. Hemorrhoids (from the Greek meaning "bleeding"), sometimes called "piles" (from the Latin meaning "a ball"), are dilated veins in the vicinity of the anus and rectum. They are similar to varicose veins of the legs, but of course are in a different location.

Hemorrhoids may be caused by a variety of conditions. Heredity probably has a role in their occurrences, as they seem to be more common in some families than in others. The human posture—being erect much of the time—puts pressure on the veins in the lower part of the body, and if the walls of these veins are weak, they will swell, resulting in varicosities in the legs and/or the rectal-anal area. Other conditions can lead to hemorrhoids in a susceptible person:

1. Chronic constipation, in which pressure is put on the rectal veins by straining at stool, can cause dilation of these thin-walled blood vessels.
2. Infection of the anal-rectal area can cause weakness of the walls of the veins and thus result in hemorrhoids.
3. Diarrhea may also weaken the walls of the rectal veins, resulting in stretching of the veins and hemorrhoids.
4. Certain occupations seem to contribute to this condition, such as those that require constant standing, especially if combined with hard manual labor. Sitting too much (presumably because exercise is necessary to maintain a brisk flow of blood through the veins) is also said to be conducive to the development of hemorrhoids.
5. Any condition which increases pressure within the abdomen is likely to cause backup of blood within the veins of the rectal area, causing them to dilate. Pregnancy, for instance, is frequently accompanied by hemorrhoids, but they usually subside after delivery of the child. Certain

medical and surgical conditions can also produce backup of the venous system with resulting hemorrhoids (and usually varicose veins of the legs). These include cirrhosis of the liver, tumors in the abdomen and digestive tract, heart failure, and others.

Symptoms of Hemorrhoids

The symptoms of hemorrhoids generally fall into three categories.

1. *Protrusion of a mass from the rectum.* This occurs especially following a bowel movement because the dilated, enlarged mass of veins is pushed out of its usual location, which is just inside the rectum, by the straining of the bowel movement. Hemorrhoids, of course, may protrude at other times as well. Simply walking, standing, coughing, and sneezing may also cause protrusion. It depends on how far advanced the hemorrhoids are, how tight the anal sphincter is, how moist they are, etc. The protrusion is usually painless, but they certainly are uncomfortable. The sufferer has no doubt that a lump is protruding from his or her rectum. It is usually accompanied by an excessive degree of mucus leakage from the rectum, a generally unpleasant set of conditions.

If hemorrhoids originate external to the anal sphincter, as they sometimes do, the dilated veins are evident under the skin, just outside the rectum. At least with the "internal" variety (those that originate within the rectum), the protrusion is intermittent. Some unlucky people have both varieties.

2. *Bleeding.* Although bleeding may occur with both internal and external hemorrhoids, this symptom is more common with internal hemorrhoids. Because pressure is placed on the weakened veins while straining at stool, bleeding is most likely to occur with a bowel movement. At times it will be noticed only by blood on the toilet tissue, at other times by bright-red blood streaking the feces, and sometimes by a gush of blood that may be quite frightening. Bleeding from hemorrhoids can be so profuse that it leads to anemia. Blood from hemorrhoids originates, of course, from the rectal area, so it is "fresh" when seen and appears bright red. Bleeding originating from higher up in the di-

Hemorrhoids

gestive tract is changed by chemicals within the gut and usually appears dark red or black. If the bleeding originates from the stomach, it may have a tarry appearance.

Hemorrhoidal bleeding is not limited to those times when a bowel movement is in progress. Should the hemorrhoid protrude, and sometimes even when it does not, bleeding may occur spontaneously while working, walking, or otherwise engaged in ordinary activities. It is particularly troublesome and embarrassing at such times. Like protrusion of the hemorrhoidal mass, bleeding is usually intermittent and there may be extensive periods of time between bleeding episodes. When it does occur, it usually lasts a few days and then subsides.

3. *Pain.* Veins are blood vessels and are therefore subject to the formation of clots within them. When this occurs, there may be considerable pain, sometimes requiring immediate surgical removal of the clot. External hemorrhoids (those outside the anal opening) are more likely to result in severe pain than those originating from within the rectum.

4. *Itching.* Some hemorrhoidal sufferers complain of itching about the rectal area. Although this is not as common as TV commercials would have us believe, it may occur when the skin about the anus is irritated by protruding hemorrhoids or by excessive mucus caused by the enlarged veins. External hemorrhoids seem more likely to be associated with itching than internal hemorrhoids. But not all anal itching is due to hemorrhoids; a variety of other conditions, such as infection, worms, and irritation from other sources, can cause anal itching, as can psychological causes.

When to See Your Doctor

All cases of anal and rectal trouble should be checked with your doctor. Let the doctor at least establish the fact that your problem is hemorrhoids. Other conditions, much more serious, can cause the same symptoms as hemorrhoids. Before you self-treat, know first what you are treating, so that you do not misdiagnose a more serious and potentially curable condition.

1. Blood in stool, whether bright red, streaked on the feces, mixed with them, dark brown, black, or in any other form or color
2. Change in bowel habit, whether it is constipation, diarrhea, or a combination of both, and whether it is intermittent or lasts for more than a few days
3. Jaundice, swelling of your legs, swelling of the abdomen, dark urine, or any other symptoms appearing more or less in conjunction with the hemorrhoids
4. Sudden onset of pain in the rectal area
5. Protrusion of hemorrhoids that cannot be replaced into the rectum, either spontaneously or by manipulation (see below)
6. Chronic irritation and/or itching of the anal area

Self-Treatment Without OTC Medication

1. Keep stools soft. This is best done by an appropriate diet (see Chapter 6); bran cereals, celery, and at least a quart of water a day. Stool softeners such as Colace and Metamucil may be needed. Regularizing bowel habits and not straining at stool are important.
2. Most protruding hemorrhoids will return to their normal position by themselves. Some will not, and require manipulation to bring them back into place. Since standing increases the pressure within the veins, simply lying down may be sufficient to correct the protruded condition. Sitz baths (another name for a hot tub bath) may relax the swelling sufficiently to allow the hemorrhoidal mass to return to its internal position.

   If protruded hemorrhoids will not return to their normal position either spontaneously or with these simple measures, it may be necessary to return them to the inside position by pushing them in with your fingers. This is best done by using a lubricant such as Vaseline, or simply soap and water, and "kneading" the swollen mass through the anal opening back into its internal position. It is not painful. The rectal area should then be thoroughly dried so the mass cannot easily slip out again. Should this type of manipulation be required more than rarely, it is time to see your doctor again and have something done about the hemorrhoids.
3. Keeping your stools soft will minimize the chances of

bleeding. However, hemorrhoids will occasionally bleed no matter what precautions are taken. If internal hemorrhoids are protruding, reduce them as described above. This will usually stop the bleeding, if it is not severe. If blood squirts out while you are having a bowel movement, it is again time to see your doctor for more definitive treatment. Chronic bleeding from hemorrhoids is a definite cause of anemia, and this can be dangerous, especially if a heart condition or other medical problem is present.
4. There are two kinds of pain: the discomfort associated with internal and external hemorrhoids, and the acute pain associated with a blood clot in one or more of the veins making up the hemorrhoidal tissue. In the former case, sitz baths may help, but if the pain is present most of the time, it is best to have an operation to relieve the condition.

For acute pain, sitz baths may also give you temporary relief, but if a bath does not relieve the pain in a few hours, your doctor should be called.

What About Surgery?

A word of reassurance about surgical treatment of hemorrhoids. First of all, there is no medicine that can *cure* hemorrhoids. Some hemorrhoids are self-limiting, such as when they occur in association with pregnancy. With the birth of the child, the major symptoms of hemorrhoids will usually disappear. In other cases, hemorrhoids are characterized by their intermittent nature. Sometimes you will not know they are present, then there may be weeks of discomfort with protrusion and possibly bleeding. Self-treatment with diet to produce soft stools and certain ointments may help you over the rough spots, but there is nothing available, either OTC or by prescription, that will effect a cure.

When the symptoms of hemorrhoids become too much of a nuisance, or when there is chronic bleeding or protrusion that will not respond to simple measures, it is time for surgery. Recent surgical techniques have greatly simplified hemorrhoidal surgery. In many cases, hemorrhoids can be removed in several outpatient visits to a doctor's office, in a minimally uncomfortable fashion. Generally, not even anesthesia is required. This is not applicable to all types of hemorrhoids; it works best with the internal type. In any event, do not be afraid to see your doctor. He will probably refer you to a specialist who can advise you of the kind of treatment best suited for your particular condition.

OTC Medications

Most of the available OTC medications for hemorrhoids are not too helpful. The best they can do is to provide a soothing ointment or cream for the swollen and irritated tissue. At times, this will decrease the general discomfort and annoyance and may allow for easier reduction of protruded internal hemorrhoids. No hemorrhoidal preparation available today is going to cure the condition, but most hemorrhoidal sufferers are thankful for little favors.

In their usual way, manufacturers of hemorrhoidal preparations have tried to be all things to all conditions. After all, they can't all have the same preparation, so they must add additional medication to the basic formula to be able to make such claims as "new and improved" and "more effective than ever." Unfortunately, most of the "additional ingredients" are useless and many are even harmful.

The basic ingredient in all hemorrhoidal preparations is a lubricant of one form or another. Vaseline will accomplish the same thing, but this is of course too simple. Cocoa butter is a popular lubricant in commercial preparations, and it is perfectly adequate (A and D Hemorrhoidal Suppositories, Wyanoids Suppositories, etc.). The most popular preparation, Preparation H, uses shark-liver oil. It sounds exotic, but there is no scientific evidence that it has much to offer over more common lubricants.

The second ingredient which most OTC medications contain is an astringent which is supposed to constrict tissue and reduce swelling. Although it is unproved that astringents do much good in the treatment of hemorrhoids, they probably do little harm.

Another popular ingredient is an antiseptic, which is supposed to have a mild anti-germ action. It does not actually kill germs, as antibiotics do, but rather it mildly retards their growth. Although probably useless in the treatment of hemorrhoids, who can complain about keeping clean?

There are two other, all-too-frequent ingredients in these preparations which have no business being there, and preparations containing them should not be used. These are local anesthetics of any kind, and vasoconstrictors, which act

Hemorrhoids

to constrict tiny blood vessels and thus retard bleeding. The difficulty with the anesthetics is that they can cause more trouble than they are worth. When used regularly, they can cause irritation and sensitization. They afford very little, if any, benefit in the treatment of hemorrhoids and because of their side effects, should not be used at all. Americaine, Eudicane, Kip, Lanacane, Nupercainal, and many others contain local anesthetics.

As far as the vasoconstrictors are concerned, they too will cause sensitization and irritation when used regularly and may do so immediately in susceptible persons. Moreover, they do little good in controlling bleeding from hemorrhoids, since hemorrhoidal bleeding is from fairly large veins and vasoconstrictors work on small arteries. Vasoconstrictors should, therefore, not be used either.

Ointments and Creams vs. Suppositories

Ointments and creams are preferable to suppositories. A suppository will not melt until placed inside the rectum and may travel quite a distance from the hemorrhoids before the ingredients are released. Furthermore, the drugs in the suppository usually get quite diluted by fluid and feces when inside the rectum, so that only low concentration of the medication actually is applied to the hemorrhoids.

When internal hemorrhoids are in place within the rectum, there is rarely need for *any* medication; it is when they protrude that help is needed, and a suppository cannot do much for hemorrhoids outside the rectum. External hemorrhoids—those normally outside the anus—will also not be helped by a suppository. The same objections apply to inserting creams or ointments inside the rectum by means of a tube or injector.

If any OTC preparation is to be used, it is best to simply apply the cream or ointment by finger to the rectal area, coating the inside of the anal sphincter with the medicine, as well.

Suggested Treatment Plan for Suspected Hemorrhoids

1. Confirm diagnosis with doctor.
2. General
   A. Regularize bowel habits (see Chapter 6).

B. Keep stools soft.
   1) Diet: bran, celery, cooked fruit and vegetables and at least a quart of water a day
   2) Colace, Metamucil, if needed
   3) No harsh cathartics
3. Protrusion of hemorrhoids
   A. Lubricant
   B. Supine position (lying down), if possible
   C. Sitz baths
   D. Manual reduction
   E. OTC medication Group I
4. Bleeding
   A. Put hemorrhoids back in position if protruding.
   B. If severe or recurrent bleeding, see doctor.
5. Pain
   A. Chronic
      1) Put back in position if protruding.
      2) Sitz baths
      3) OTC medication Group I
   B. Acute
      1) Sitz baths
      2) Call doctor.
6. Itching
   A. Confirm diagnosis with doctor.
   B. Sitz baths
   C. OTC medication Group I
   D. Prescription medicine containing cortisone is usually more effective than OTC preparations.

OTC Hemorrhoidal Preparations

GROUP I
Acceptable

Examples of preparations containing only a lubricant and/or antiseptic and/or astringent (*creams and ointments are preferred to suppositories*):

Name	Form	Approximate Cost
A and D Hemorrhoidal Suppositories	Suppositories #12	for $1.82
Anusol	Ointment 1 oz.	for 1.80
	Suppositories #12	for 2.23
Calmol 4	Suppositories #12	for 1.99

Dorana	Suppositories	#12	for	1.98
Preparation H	Ointment	1 oz.	for	1.79
	Suppositories	#12	for	2.23
Tucks cream, ointment	Ointment	40 gm	for	1.85
	Cream	40 gm	for	1.85
Vaseline Hemorr-Aid	Ointment	1 oz.	for	1.09
Vaseline Petroleum Jelly	Jelly	7½ oz.	for	.99*

GROUP II
Unacceptable

These preparations contain local anesthetics and/or vasoconstrictors.

Name	Form
A-Caine	Ointment
Americaine	Suppositories
	Ointment
Diothane	Ointment
Eudicane	Suppositories
Hemor-Rid Rectal Ointment	Ointment
Kip Hemorrhoid Relief	Ointment
	Suppositories
Lanacane Creme	Cream
Nupercainal	Ointment
	Suppositories
Pazo	Ointment
	Suppositories
Perifoam	Aerosol
PNS	Suppositories
Rectalgan	Liquid
Rectal Medicone	Suppositories
	Ointment (unguent)
Wyanoids	Ointment
	Suppositories

* Best buy in group.

Chapter 8

Acne and Other Skin Problems

Treatment of skin problems accounts for a major share of the OTC drug market. Throughout this book, the limited effectiveness of many OTC drugs has been emphasized. However with skin diseases, the situation is quite different. Because the medication is applied *to* the skin and not taken internally, it is possible to purchase relatively effective medicines for simple skin difficulties. In many instances, it is the same medication your doctor would prescribe, although it may be packaged somewhat differently. This is not to say that in severe cases your doctor does not have more potent medication (and other treatment methods) than those available to the public he has. But for mild skin problems, self-treatment is often very effective.

Acne

Acne is characterized by pimples and blackheads, usually beginning about the time of puberty and most commonly visible over the face and forehead. In more advanced cases, acne can spread to the neck, chest, back, and upper arms. The pimples and blackheads are caused by plugging of tiny oil (sebaceous) glands in the skin. These glands normally discharge their contents into the lumen of hair shafts within the skin. The oil-like material (sebum) manufactured in the sebaceous glands lubricates the hair shafts and spreads onto the surface of the skin. When the openings of these hair follicles or "pores" become clogged due to overgrowth of skin, or excessively thick sebum, the oil-like material manufactured within the glands will "dam up" behind the obstruction. When the secretions accumulate in this fashion, they turn into a waxy substance, causing the pores to bulge. This is the simple pimple or "whitehead." When the opening of the pore is not completely closed and thus slightly exposed to air, the

Acne and Other Skin Problems

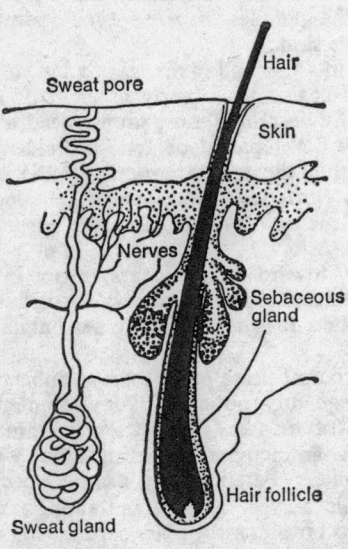

FIGURE 4
Skin

waxy substance "oxidizes" and turns black, much as a sliced apple left in air will do. This is the "blackhead" and is not simply a dirty pimple. Whiteheads and blackheads are the major components of simple acne. The disease may become more complicated, however, if the whiteheads or blackheads become infected, as they frequently do. In even more advanced cases, the pimples may eventually result in scarring and pitting of the skin.

Acne occurs in almost all humans, to a lesser or greater extent, sometimes beginning as early as eight or nine years of age, but generally becoming most pronounced about the time of puberty. The development of acne coincides with hormonal changes within the body, particularly the production of male hormones (girls also produce a slight amount of male hormone). Hormonal changes, however, are not the sole cause of acne.

The tendency toward acne appears to run in families and may even be related, in some cases, to diet, exercise, and other health habits. It is *not* related to sex habits such as masturbation.

Acne may occur at times other than at puberty. Menstruating women frequently notice the development of pimples about the time of menses. In addition, certain women may develop acne (or an increase in existing acne) with the use of birth-control pills. (Paradoxically, some special kinds of birth-control pills are very effective in treating acne.)

In addition to birth-control pills, certain other medications may cause acne, particularly cortisone or cortisonelike drugs such as prednisone, Decadron, etc.

A few diseases, especially those associated with hormonal abnormalities, may cause skin eruptions, so if acne develops in the adult, it is important to check with the doctor to be certain that no underlying medical condition is present.

Some women develop facial pimples as a result of cosmetics. The cosmetics either cause an allergic reaction, or act to plug up the pores, preventing the flow of oils and resulting in acne.

Most cases of "naturally" occurring acne are relatively mild. The problem comes and goes during adolescence and sometimes into early adulthood. By the mid-twenties, most skins have cleared up. However, those with persistent and severe cases of acne should be treated by a physician and/or skin specialist without relying on home remedies, so that pitting and scarring may be avoided. One study of over 1,000 high school students with acne showed that about 2 percent had a severe form of the skin problem, requiring expert medical attention.

Treatment of Simple Acne

For simple acne (mild cases without accompanying infection), treatment should be directed at keeping the skin clean and using a mild abrasive to "peel" the outer layer of skin so that the pores will open to the surface.

Diet should be well balanced and table salt without iodine (which may increase the production of skin oil) should be used. Excessive sweets should be avoided and, if overweight, a weight reduction diet should be instituted.

The use of medicated creams and lotions which will "peel" the skin will also help open the pores and allow for free flow of the natural skin oils.

In addition, it is well known that sunshine markedly aids the regression of acne. Either natural sunshine or a sun lamp at home can be of considerable help.

High doses of vitamin A have recently been advocated for treatment of acne, but this is still experimental and, if used, should be initiated by a physician.

Suggested Treatment Program for Simple Acne

1. Do not pick pimples. Keep hands off your face. Large whiteheads or blackheads that are not infected should be "expressed," but this is best done by your doctor, who will demonstrate the proper technique. Casual picking at your face will only spread the acne, and may cause pitting of the skin.
2. Diet should be well balanced, but low in sweets. Table salt without iodine should be used. If overweight, go on a reducing diet.
3. Get as much natural sunshine as possible. In winter, the use of a sun lamp may be used. Start with one minute a day and build up slowly to ten minutes a day. Proper timing is indicated by slight facial redness persisting through

the following day. Be certain that someone else is at home when using the lamp. Do not overuse and do not put any lotions or medicines on face while sunning. Cover eyes with dark or moist pads when exposed to either sun or sun lamp.
4. Use no cosmetics, creams, etc. without first checking with your doctor.
5. Use plain soap and warm water at least twice a day on the affected areas. Abrasive soaps (Brasivol, fine, medium, or rough; Pernox) are generally more effective but may be irritating to some users. However, they are worth a try. Begin with Brasivol, fine, twice a day. Scrub on face (and other affected areas) for 30 seconds to one minute, until the skin begins to hurt slightly. If this treatment is tolerated without excessive irritation for a few weeks, you may progress to medium or rough textures of the soap. If the abrasive soaps cannot be used, plain, unmedicated hand soaps will do. Do not use any special "acne soaps" or "skin cleaners" (Noxzema Skin Cream, etc.) as they have little to offer over plain soap.
6. Use a drying lotion or cream containing benzoyl peroxide, sulfur, resorcinol, and/or salicylic acid. Products containing benzoyl peroxide (Benoxyl, Oxy-5, etc.) are the strongest. Intermediate in strength are the preparations containing at least 2 percent sulfur (Acne, Acne-Dome, etc.), with or without resorcinol. The least effective are those containing only resorcinol and salicylic acid.

For moderate to severe acne, the benzoyl products should be used first. When the skin condition is brought under control or if the acne is mild to begin with, sulfur-containing products can be used.

These preparations should be applied both during the day and at night, in order to maintain *mild* dryness and redness. If there is discomfort, you have used too much. For special daytime use, tinted creams may be used such as Acnomel, Fostril, etc.
7. Acne is a chronic problem and must be kept after for years or it will be certain to return.
8. If these measures are not effective in alleviating acne, your physician should take over. He may wish to use antibiotics, hormone treatment, and other drugs and procedures which may be more effective.

Acne and Other Skin Problems

Drying Agents for Acne

GROUP I
Strongest
These contain benzoyl peroxide.

Name	Form	Approximate Cost
Benoxyl-5	Lotion	1 oz. for $3.20
Dry and Clear W/N-12	Lotion	2 oz. for 3.10
Loroxide	Lotion	25 gm. for 3.40
Oxy-5	Lotion	1 oz. for 2.49
Pan-Oxyl-5	Gel	2 oz. for 2.94*
Persadox	Lotion, cream	1 oz. for 3.00
Vanoxide	Lotion	25 gm. for 3.00

GROUP II
Intermediate Strength
These contain sulfur.

Name	Form	Approximate Cost
Acne-Aid	Cream	1.8 oz. for $2.25
Acnederm	Lotion	2 oz. for 1.96
Acne-Dome	Cream	1 oz. for 3.29
Acnomel	Cream	1 oz. for 1.98
	Cake	1 oz. for 1.98
Cenac	Lotion	2 oz. for 2.10
Clearasil	Stick	⅛ oz. for 1.29
Clearasil Regular Tinted	Cream	1.2 oz. for 1.85
Clearasil Vanishing Formula	Cream	1.2 oz. for 1.85
Contrablem	Gel	1 oz. for 2.50
Fostex	Cream	4½ oz. for 2.95
	Liquid	5 oz. for 2.55*
Fostril	Cream	1 oz. for 2.39
Klaron	Lotion	2 oz. for 2.85
Liquimat	Lotion	1.5 oz. for 2.00
pHisoAc	Cream	1½ oz. for 1.89
piSec	Cream	1½ oz. for 2.85
Resulin	Lotion	4 oz. for 2.45

* Best buy(s) in group.

Rezamid	Lotion, cream	2 oz. for	2.65
Xerac	Gel	1½ oz. for	2.95

GROUP III
Lesser Strength
These contain resorcinol and/or salicylic acid.

Name	Form	Approximate Cost	
Acnesarb	Solution	4 oz. for	$1.57*
Komed Regular	Lotion	1¾ oz. for	2.52
Microsyn	Lotion	2 oz. for	2.52
Tackle	Clear Gel	2 oz. for	1.89

GROUP IV
Not Recommended

Not recommended due to lack of effective ingredients or insufficient concentrations of otherwise effective ingredients

Ice-O-Derm
Ionax
Jergens Clear Complexion Gel
Komed Mild
Lotioblanc
Medicated Face Conditioner (MFC)
Noxzema Skin Cream
pHisoDerm Medicated Liquid
Pro-Blem
Pronac
Sebacide
Seba-Nil
Stri-Dex Medicated Pads
Teenac
Therapads Plus
Ting

---

* Best buy in group.

Dandruff

Dandruff is one form of a generalized skin condition known as seborrheic dermatitis, sometimes referred to as seborrhea. It is a scaling eruption associated with redness and frequently with itching. Seborrhea is most often found on the scalp and is then referred to as dandruff. However, it may also be present on the face, eyebrows and eyelids, ears, behind the ears, chest, under the arms, back, around the navel, and sometimes surrounding the genital organs.

The cause is not known. It may occur at any age, including infants ("cradle cap"). Seborrheic dermatitis may progress from its usual mild state to a severe skin problem with crusting and secondary infection requiring considerable medical skill to treat effectively. Some diseases, particularly Parkinson's disease, have a high incidence of seborrhea. There is also a tendency to have dandruff if acne is present. Perhaps this indicates that dandruff has a relation to excessive oil secretions, but this is not certain. The severe forms of dandruff are associated with early baldness in men.

Treatment of Dandruff

The basic treatment of dandruff is to shampoo the scalp and hair two or three times a week with medicated shampoos. Many of the OTC shampoos contain the same medication a physician would recommend and usually produce satisfactory results. If seborrhea extends beyond the hair to include face, ears, and other skin areas, the same OTC hair shampoo may be tried on the skin. If relief is not forthcoming in a few weeks, a physician should be consulted.

Group I contains primarily antiseptic solutions rather than specific anti-dandruff medication, but they are sometimes quite effective and may be tried before those in Group II, especially if a "milder" preparation is desired, or if the dandruff problem is not severe.

Any of the shampoos listed in Group II is medically satisfactory and all will yield approximately equivalent results. The choice is made on the basis of personal preference and price. At times, certain shampoos seem to work better for some persons than for others, but this is unpredictable. Those preparations containing tar may stain blond or gray hair and are listed separately in Group III.

Once dandruff is brought under control, it will probably return unless the shampooing is continued at least once a week. In some instances, the effectiveness of the shampoo that originally helped wears off, and another brand must be substituted. This should be no problem since there are many on the OTC market from which to choose.

As usual, if dandruff or seborrheic skin lesions are not significantly relieved with OTC preparations in a few weeks, see your doctor. You may be attempting to treat skin problems other than seborrheic dermatitis. Psoriasis is the skin problem most likely to be confused with seborrhea, whether it be on the scalp or other areas of the body.

Dandruff Preparations

GROUP I
Mild Preparations

Examples of mild shampoos without specific dandruff medication

Name	Approximate Cost
Betadine Shampoo	4 oz. for $1.98
Dandricide Shampoo	4 oz. for 2.25
Double Danderine	10 oz. for 1.39*
Drest	3½ oz. for 1.95
Monique Dandruff Control Shampoo and Rinse	8 oz. for 2.50
Ogilvie Anti-Dandruff Shampoo	8 oz. for 2.25
Rinse Away Shampoo	3 oz. for 1.09
Scadan	4 oz. for 3.30
Seret	8 oz. for 3.00
Sulfur-8 Shampoo	6 oz. for 1.19
Tame Creme Rinse	4 oz. for 0.90
Thylox PDC	6 oz. for 1.98
Top Brass Cream	4 oz. for 1.00
Zincon	4 oz. for 2.10
ZP-11	3.5 oz. for 1.50

* Best buy in group.

GROUP II
Anti-Dandruff Preparations

Examples of shampoos containing anti-dandruff medication

Name	Form	Approximate Cost
Breck One Dandruff Shampoo		6 oz. for $2.00
Denorex Shampoo		4 oz. for 2.09
Enden Shampoo		5 oz. for 1.09
Fomac Cream Cleanser		3½ oz. for 1.95
Fostex Cake Bar		3¾ oz. for 1.39
Head & Shoulders		4 oz. for 1.39
		4 oz. for 0.90
Ionil		4 oz. for 2.55
Ionil T		4 oz. for 2.85
Klaron Lotion		2 oz. for 1.90
Meted Shampoo		4 oz. for 2.35
Meted 2 Shampoo		4 oz. for 2.35
pHisoDan		5 oz. for 2.29
Resorcitate		8 oz. for 2.45
Rezamid Shampoo		6 oz. for 2.40
Sebaveen		4 oz. for 2.52
Sebulex		4 oz. for 2.75
		4 oz. for 2.29
Selenium Blue		8 oz. for 3.22
Selenium Sulfide (various manufacturers—Moore, Pharmecon, etc.)		4 oz. for 1.33
Selsun Blue		4 oz. for 2.29
Sulfur-8 Conditioner		4 oz. for 1.99
Vanseb		3 oz. for 2.31

GROUP III
Tar-Containing Preparations

All the following contain tar, which may stain blond or gray hair.

Alma Tar
Mazon Shampoo
Pragmatar

Psorex
Sebutone
Tegrin Shampoo
Tentrax
Vanseb-T Tar
Zetar

Cold Sores, Fever Blisters, Herpes Simplex, and Canker Sores

These are all names for the same condition. It is a recurrent problem caused by a specific virus or viruses. It produces small blisters which usually itch. They are most commonly found on the lips, face, and genital areas. It sometimes occurs on the eye, which, in some cases, can lead to blindness. When it occurs in the newborn child, it can be a serious disease.

The virus can be spread from person to person through close contact. Thus, kissing (if the sore is present on the lips) or sexual intercourse (if present in the genital area) should be avoided during the course of the disease.

In mild cases the use of rubbing alcohol and OTC preparations listed in Groups I or II may be of some help. The lesions will spontaneously disappear in a week or two but they frequently recur in the same location, sometimes years after the initial infection. This is so because the virus may lie dormant in the skin and be activated at a later time by an upper respiratory infection, trauma, excessive exposure to sun, or other stimuli.

In any but the mildest cases, a physician should be consulted as he can use more potent medication than is available OTC.

OTC Preparations for Cold Sores

There are basically two types of OTC preparations available for the treatment of simple cold sores. The first contains an astringent such as phenol which acts to tighten or contract the tissue to which it is applied and thus, it is believed, promote healing. Group I lists the OTC preparations containing astringents and other miscellaneous drugs promoted for cold sores.

The second group of OTC products sold for cold sores contains a local anesthetic, usually benzocaine, combined with phenol and other medications found in Group I. Except for the few persons who may be sensitive to local anesthetics, the medicines are harmless if not used to excess. It is best to try one of the preparations in Group I first and, if relief is insufficient, try one with a local anesthetic listed in Group II. The products listed within each group are of approximately equal effectiveness (or lack thereof).

OTC Preparations for Cold Sores

GROUP I
Examples of Astringents and Miscellaneous Medicines

Name	Form	Approximate Cost
Blistaid	Lotion	0.5 oz. for $0.56
Blister Klear	Stick	0.1 oz. for 0.59
Blistex	Ointment	0.42 oz. for 1.19
Campho-Phenique	Liquid	1.0 oz. for 0.79*
Cankaid	Liquid	0.75 oz. for 2.10

GROUP II
Examples of Preparations Containing Local Anesthetics

Name	Form	Approximate Cost
Ambesol	Liquid	0.31 oz. for $1.50
Bio-Stik	Stick	0.1 oz. for 1.49
Dalidyne	Liquid, cream	0.25 oz. for 1.29
Solarcaine Lip Balm	Salve	1.0 oz. for 0.99*
Tanac	Stick, liquid	0.5 oz. for 1.49

Skin Problems Which Should Not Be Self-Treated with OTC Drugs

1. *Psoriasis.* This disease is often confused with seborrhea or dandruff. Its most noticeable symptom is scaling. Itching

---
* Best buy(s) in group.

occurs in about 20 percent of patients with this problem. It is occasionally accompanied by arthritis. The scaling may be localized to the scalp, but almost any other part of the body may be involved. When the scaling is generalized, it is most commonly present over the elbows and knees.

Psoriasis is a chronic disease, but modern treatment is quite effective in most cases. However, the best medications for this condition must be prescribed by physicians. In very mild cases, some of the OTC preparations may be partially effective, but because of the complexity of the disease, treatment is best begun by a professional.

2. *Eczema.* From the medical viewpoint, "eczema" is a term used to describe a group of diseases, rather than a single entity. The common denominator to these diseases is some form of allergic reaction expressed as a skin disorder. It may occur in infancy (infantile eczema) or in adults. It may be due to an allergy to foods, soaps, plants (poison oak or ivy), or other agents with which we may come in contact. It may be mild or severe. In adults the lesions are frequently found in the area of contact of the offending irritant (hands, etc.) and/or the inner portion of the elbows and knees. In addition to the rash, itching is a very prominent symptom and many eczema sufferers get into further difficulty because of scratching and the secondary infection which this causes.

Treatment is generally effective, but should be initiated and supervised by a physician.

Chapter 9

Burns and Sunburn

Although the skin provides an amazingly efficient protective cover for our bodies it is sometimes damaged by chemical and/or physical agents. Excessive heat is perhaps the most common cause of such damage. It makes relatively little difference what the source of the heat is; if it rises above a certain point for a sufficient time, a burn will result. As far as injury to the skin is concerned, the damage is the same whether the burn is a result of fire, a hot stove, or the sun. Only the extent and severity of the burn will differ.

Types of Burns (Including Sunburn)

1. *First-degree burns.* This is the mildest form of burn. The usual sunburn and cooking accidents most often fall into this category. The skin becomes red, painful, and sometimes swollen. There is no break in the skin and no blisters develop.

2. *Second-degree burns.* This is still a superficial burn in that only the outermost layers of the skin are involved. As with first-degree burns, the skin becomes red and painful, but with second-degree burns, swelling is more likely to occur. The most characteristic feature of second-degree burns, however, is the development of blisters. In the healing stages, there will be regrowth of new skin.

3. *Third-degree burns.* This is the most serious form of burn and is seen in fire victims and some chemical burns. It is a deep burn and most or all of the skin thickness is injured. When third-degree burns are present over a large portion of the body, it can be fatal. In the past few years special "burn centers" have been established in a number of hospi-

tals around the country. This has resulted in a significant reduction of deaths from third-degree burns.

Treatment of First-Degree Burns

First-degree burns may be treated at home.

1. Apply cold compresses or ice packs or immerse the affected portion of the body in cold tapwater. This will usually produce relief of pain and may help prevent more extensive skin injury. The application of cold should be maintained until the area is free of pain, which may take up to an hour. The sooner after the burn exposure this treatment is begun, the better the results.
2. No further treatment is usually needed for first-degree burns. However, if pain should persist, plain aspirin, two or three tablets with a full glass of water or with food, three or four times a day will usually provide sufficient relief. If aspirin cannot be tolerated, acetaminophen (Tylenol, etc.) may be substituted in the same dosage.
3. Local anesthetics are usually not necessary for first-degree burns. However, when the burns are extensive and relatively severe, such as with a severe sunburn, local anesthetics may afford additional relief, especially during the night when pain is frequently exaggerated. There are a wide variety of local anesthetics available OTC. However, the only preparations that are effective are ones containing over 5 percent benzocaine (or a similar local anesthetic), and preferably 20 percent. Americaine is the most popular OTC local anesthetic with this high concentration of drug. Burntame spray and TegaCaine aerosol also contain 20 percent benzocaine. Kip spray contains 10 percent benzocaine but none of the other popular products for this purpose contains sufficient local anesthetic to be effective.

    On the negative side of local anesthetics is the fact that skin sensitization occurs with their use in some persons. Should this occur, it will add to the discomfort and pain of the existing burn. If you wish to use a local anesthetic, the best choice would be Americaine ointment or spray, and first test an *un*involved portion of your body. If there is no reaction in 30 minutes, you may apply it to the burn.
4. *Do not* use home remedies such as butter or lard.

Burns and Sunburn

5. *Do not* use antibiotic creams, ointments, or sprays without a doctor's advice.

Treatment of Second-Degree Burns

Second-degree burns include severe sunburns. Second-degree burns covering only small areas of the body (the tip of the finger, for instance) may be treated at home. If there is more extensive damage, it should be treated by a doctor.

1. The same procedures for the treatment of first-degree burns apply here (in fact, prompt "cold" treatment of the burn may prevent blistering). The major difference is the care of the blisters, which are the hallmark of the second-degree burn. These are best treated with salt-water compresses for 30 to 60 minutes, three or four times a day. Immerse a towel in salt water made up of two tablespoons of table salt to a quart of cold tap water, and keep the dressing continuously wet.
2. Aspirin by mouth (as above), Americaine, etc. and sometimes a mild, soothing ointment (Vaseline) should be sufficient.
3. If extensive areas of the body are burned, or if small burns become infected (which does *not* often happen with second-degree burns), professional help must be sought.
4. Severe sunburns (or burns from a sun lamp) can be greatly helped if very early treatment with cortisone is instituted. This, of course, will be done only by your physician and only in severe cases.

Treatment of Third-Degree Burns

Third-degree burns are emergency situations and the closest emergency room, hospital, or physician should be consulted, particularly if the burn is extensive.

1. Third-degree burns are usually not as painful as first- or second-degree burns (because the nerve endings in the skin have also been destroyed) and emergency treatment consists of gentle washing of the involved area with tepid

soapy water. Ivory or other "gentle" soap may be used until a physician can be consulted.
2. *Do not* put any ointments, creams, anesthetics, antibiotics, or other medications on the burn.

Prevention of Sunburn

It is much easier to prevent sunburn than to treat it. The ultimate prevention is simply to stay out of the sun. Now that we have dispensed with this impractical advice, we can consider the OTC products that are available which will allow us the pleasures of the sun with minimal after-effects.

There are two types of products sold for this purpose: sunshades and sunscreens (both of the chemical variety).

Sunshades are opaque substances which act to prevent the sun from reaching the skin. They simply block out all or most of the sun's rays. Sunshades are most often used by sun-worshippers on the nose and lips. Zinc oxide, a white paste available in all drugstores, is the cheapest and most effective preparation for this purpose. A-Fil and Solar Cream are similar in effect (they contain titanium dioxide) but are prepackaged and therefore more costly, though not more effective.

*Sunscreen*s include the usual sun lotions, creams, sprays, etc. which are so widely advertised and marketed. Sunscreens differ from sunshade products in that the former allow some of the sun's rays to reach the skin, permitting a mild sunburn and tanning, but block out the more harmful rays, thus preventing extensive sunburn.

The most effective sunscreens contain the chemical para-aminobenzoic acid (PABA), in an alcohol base. Researchers at Harvard Medical School showed that in addition to being the most effective sunscreen available, it also had the added benefit of being relatively resistant to removal by swimming or perspiration. The single disadvantage to this chemical is that it may produce a permanent yellow stain on light-colored clothing, especially cotton. Also, like all chemicals, these preparations may be irritating to the skin of some users.

These sunscreens (Pabanal, PreSun, etc.) should be applied about an hour before intended exposure for best results. It is important to remember that although these products are more resistant than most to being washing off, they should usually be reapplied after swimming.

Somewhat less effective, but still better than most sunscreens, are those that utilize a "first cousin" to PABA (Block Out, Pabafilm, Sea & Ski, etc.).

Even less effective, but also better than the run-of-the-mill suntan products, are those containing another chemical, benzophenone (Solbar, Uval). These preparations wash off more easily than the PABA preparations, but they do have the advantage of being less sensitizing to the skin than PABA products. Should the PABA preparations produce any irritation of the skin, Solbar or Uval should be tried.

Adverse Effects of Excessive Sun Exposure

1. Dizziness, chills, nausea, prostration, and dehydration may occur in extreme cases of excessive sun exposure. The condition is usually termed "heat stroke" or "sun sickness." The full syndrome occurs only rarely in temperate climates, but some of the symptoms may occur with overzealous sunbathers. If mild, the symptoms will pass spontaneously when retiring to a cooler environment and drinking sufficient fluids. In more severe cases, a doctor should be consulted.
2. Certain diseases are intensified by exposure to sunlight. These include herpes simplex (fever blister, cold sore), lupus erythematosus, and porphyria. Pregnant women are also more sensitive to the effects of sun exposure.
3. There are many drugs that will produce adverse reactions when activated by excessive exposure to sunlight. These reactions may result in skin difficulties such as blisters, redness, "hives," peeling, etc. If you are taking *any* prescription drug, ask your doctor what possible effect prolonged sun exposure might have before you try to turn yourself into a beet. Although there are additional drugs that might produce "photosensitization" with sun exposure in sensitive persons, some of the more common drugs that are likely to react with a skin reaction to sun exposure are specified in the following list.

Photosensitizing Drugs

Antibiotics: Aureomycin, Declomycin, Terramycin
Anti-diabetic medications: Diabinese, Orinase
Anti-fungal medications: Fulvicin, Griseofulvin
Antihistamines: Trilafon, Phenergan
Anti-seizure medications: Dilantin, Tridione, Tegretol
Arthritis medication: Butazolidin
Diuretics: Diuril, Hydrodiuril, Esidrix
Heart medication: Dilantin
High-blood-pressure medications: Reserpine, Serpasil
Mood elevators for depression: Tofranil, Nopramin, Pertofrane
Tranquilizers: Thorazine, Aventyl, Compazine, Sparine, Stelazine
Urinary-tract-infection drugs: Azo Gantrisin, Gantrisin, NegGram

OTC Preparations for Treatment of Burns and Sunburn

GROUP I
Recommended

A. Local anesthetics

Name	Form	Approximate Cost
Americaine	Ointment	1 oz. for $1.65
	Spray	1 oz. for 1.83
Burntame Spray	Spray	3½ oz. for 2.98
Kip Sunburn Spray	Aerosol	4 oz. for 1.98
Tega-Caine	Aerosol	5½ oz. for 2.52

B. Soothing creams

Name	Form	Approximate Cost
Johnson & Johnson First Aid Cream	Cream	2½ oz. for $2.14
	Ointment	1¼ oz. for 1.10
Noxzema Medicated Skin Cream	Cream	4 oz. for 1.35
Resinol	Ointment	3½ oz. for 2.25
Unguentine Ointment "Original Formula"	Ointment	1 oz. for 1.19

Vaseline Carbolated Petroleum Jelly	Ointment	3¾ oz. for	0.99
Vaseline Pure Petroleum Jelly	Gel	3¾ oz. for	0.79*

* Best buy in group.

GROUP II
Not Recommended

A. Examples of preparations that are ineffective and/or contain insufficient medication

Burn-a-lay
Kip First Aid Spray
Kip Moisturizing Lotion
Medicone Dressing Cream
Noxzema Sunburn Spray
Nupercainal
Pontocaine
Solarcaine
Unguentine Plus
Unguentine Spray

B. Examples of preparations containing antibiotics

Bacimycin
Clean 'N Treat
Myotrain
Spectrocin
Terramycin Ointment

OTC Preparations for Prevention of Sunburn: Sunscreens

GROUP I
Recommended

Examples of PABA preparations

Name	*Approximate Cost*
PABAGEL	4 oz. for $3.00

Pabanol	4 oz. for	2.52
Paba-Tan	4 oz. for	1.89*
PreSun	4 oz. for	3.35
Super Shade Lotion by Coppertone	4 oz. for	3.10

GROUP II
Acceptable

A. Examples of PABA-like preparations

Name	Approximate Cost
Block Out	4 oz. for $3.00
Pabafilm	4 oz. for 3.30
Sea & Ski	4 oz. for 2.00
Snootie	1 oz. for 0.99
Sure Tan	8 oz. for 2.75
Swedish Tanning Secret Lotion	4 oz. for 1.75
Oil	4 oz. for 1.75
Uval Sun'n Wind Stick	0.16 oz. for 0.85

B. Examples of benzophenone preparations

Name	Approximate Cost
Solbar	2½ oz. for $3.25
Uval Sun Screen Lotion	75 gm for 3.20

GROUP III
Not Recommended

These products offer no significant protection against sunburn.

Baby oil
Cocoa butter
Coconut oil
Mineral oil
Olive oil

---

* Best buy in group.

OTC Preparations for Prevention of Sunburn: Sunshades

GROUP I
Recommended

Name	*Approximate Cost*
Zinc oxide (various manufacturers)	1 oz. for $0.59

GROUP II
Acceptable

Name	*Approximate Cost*
A-Fil Cream	1.5 oz. for $1.95
Solar Cream (also contains PABA)	1 oz. for 3.15

Chapter 10

Poison Ivy
(Poison Oak and Poison Sumac)

Poison ivy, poison oak, and poison sumac belong to a single family of plants (*Rhus* plants) which has over 400 members, many of which are poisonous to man. Poison ivy is especially prevalent in the northeastern United States and adjacent southeastern Canada. It is not present in the coastal area of the Pacific northwest, but poison oak makes up for the lack of poison ivy in that region. From a medical viewpoint, the treatment of all plant poisons which produce their ill effects by direct contact with the skin is the same. In fact, it is very similar to the treatment of other "contact" dermatoses such as allergic reactions to soaps, metals, hair dyes, deodorants, etc.

Poison ivy (and the other poisonous plant contacts) is basically an allergic reaction to the oils of the plant. Almost everyone is susceptible, although children from three to late teens are particularly prone to develop the skin reaction when in contact with the poisonous plant. Peak incidence of poison ivy is in the spring, but it may occur at any time of the year. Depending on the extent of the exposure, and how many previous contacts there have been, the time lag between plant contact and the development of the skin rash is between 12 hours and two weeks. The more frequently prior contacts have occurred, the less the "incubation period." The rash usually lasts between two and three weeks.

The first symptom is itching, sometimes becoming very intense. This is quickly followed by patches or streaks of reddened skin, and blisters. Scratch marks usually add to the skin problems and can produce infection. Streaks or patches of redness are a sign of plant poisoning and will help distinguish it from insect bites, heat rash, etc. Because often the victim is unaware of the plant contact, and because it may take a long time for the rash to develop (especially if this is the first contact), it is sometimes difficult to determine the cause of the itching. If you have been in a wooded area within the last two weeks, plant poisoning should be suspected.

Suggested Treatment of Poison Ivy, Poison Oak, and Poison Sumac

1. *Immediate treatment.* Wash the involved areas with soap and water as soon after exposure as possible. Unfortunately, in most cases this cannot be accomplished soon enough to do much good, but it may help.

2. *Mild cases*
   A. Itching can be partially controlled by application of cold water or Burow's solution compresses for 20 to 30 minutes, four to six times a day, followed by an application of calamine lotion. Burow's solution can be bought from the pharmacy without prescription or made up by dissolving one Domeboro tablet (Bur-veen and Bluboro are similar products) in 1 pint of water.
   B. Aveeno bath (one cup to a tub of water) is also soothing.
   C. If itching is severe, a very *hot* tub bath or shower may help temporarily.
   D. Plain aspirin, two or three tablets, three or four times a day with a full glass of water or with meals, may afford significant relief from the itching. This is particularly worthwhile before retiring.
   E. An OTC sleep-aid (see Chapter 16) may also help keep you from scratching the night away.

3. *Severe cases.* See your physician if the following applies:
   A. Large areas of body involved
   B. Face involved
   C. Eyes reddened and/or swollen
   D. Infection present
   E. Itching not controlled by aspirin.

Your physician can prescribe ointments containing cortisone, but even more effective are shots or the oral use of cortisonelike agents. This type of treatment has been extremely effective in reducing the miseries of plant poisoning.

OTC Preparations for Poison Ivy, Poison Oak, and Poison Sumac

Most OTC products for poison ivy contain an antihistamine and a low-dose local anesthetic, as well as a soothing lotion such as calamine. The concentration of the local anesthetic is too low to do much good, and the local application of antihistamines to control itching has never been shown to be worthwhile. When used for poison ivy, they can only compound the difficulties in susceptible persons. The calamine lotion in poison-ivy preparations will help most mild cases, but it is more sensible, safer, and certainly cheaper to buy the least expensive calamine lotion available without the added ingredients.

OTC Preparations for Poison Ivy, Poison Oak, and Poison Sumac

GROUP I
Recommended

A. Burow's solution

Name	Approximate Cost
Burow's solution (various manufacturers)	16 oz. for $1.27*
Bluboro Powder	12 packets for 2.10
Bur-veen Powder	6 packets for 1.46
Domeboro Tablets or Powder	12 packets for 2.10

B. Calamine lotion

Calamine lotion (various manufacturers)	4 oz. for $0.70*
Comfortine ointment	4 oz. for 2.25
CZO Lotion	3 oz. for 1.12

C. Miscellaneous

Aveeno Powder	1 lb. for $2.73

* Best buy(s) in group.

GROUP II
Not Recommended

Examples of preparations containing unnecessary and/or ineffective ingredients

Name	Comment
Caladryl	Antihistamine
Calamatum Spray, Ointment & Lotion	Local anesthetic
Dalicote	Antihistamine
Dri-Toxen	Antihistamine
Ivarest	Local anesthetic, Antihistamine
Poison Ivy Cream	Local anesthetic, Antihistamine
Pontocaine Cream, Ointment	Local anesthetic
Rhuli Cream, Spray and Rhulihist	Local anesthetic
Ziradryl	Antihistamine

Chapter 11

Eye Problems

The eye is a complicated and, of course, extremely important organ of our body. The part of our eye we can inspect is just the tip of the iceberg. Most of the "working" portion of the eye is encased within the facial bones, which provide important protection for this delicate organ (see the illustration). Looking at the portion of the eye that is exposed, we see (from the periphery to the center) the white material (sclera), surrounding a colored ring (iris), in the center of which is a dark circle (pupil), through which the light rays pass to the back of the eye. Over the colored ring and dark circle (iris and pupil) is a transparent membrane (cornea) which melds into the white sclera. Covering all these parts, and extending onto the inner surface of both the lower and upper eyelids, is a thin membrane called the conjunctiva. This is like a cellophane or other transparent membrane which covers the entire exposed surface of the eyeball. It is this protective covering, the conjunctiva, that is usually affected by superficial eye problems, and for which there is such a variety of OTC medicine available.

As with almost all medical problems, the symptoms may be trivial or they may represent a serious disease. The exposed portion of the eye has only a limited number of ways it can react to injury, and therefore the same symptoms may appear whether there is dust in the eye or whether a serious infection is present. It may be very difficult for the nonprofessional observer (and sometimes for the expert) to make this distinction by casual observation. The major ways in which the conjunctiva will react to harmful stimuli, whether the cause is serious or inconsequential, are redness (due to enlargement of the blood vessels within the conjunctiva), tearing, discharge, dryness, discomfort, or burning. Severe pain is not usually part of conjunctival disease and if present, it suggests involvement of deeper structures, such as the cornea.

**FIGURE 5
The Eye**

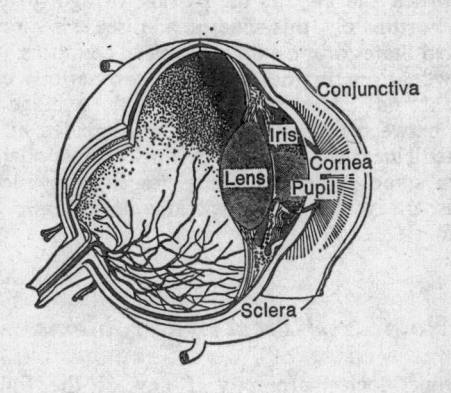

As far as OTC treatment of eye problems is concerned, one should be reasonably certain that the problem is conjunctival, and not due to involvement of deeper structures. Although this is the first consideration, it is certainly not the last, since even conjunctival diseases may be very serious. In fact, the world's most common casue of blindness is due to a viral infection of the conjunctiva (trachoma), which spreads to the cornea and impairs the passage of light to the back of the eye. Fortunately, this widespread disease is rarely found in the United States or most other Western countries.

However, even in the United States, serious conjunctival diseases are not infrequent. How does the average person distinguish between problems that may be treated at home with OTC medicines and those requiring professional attention? Here are some guidelines. They are certainly not infallible and it is always best to check any uncertainties with your physician.

When Not to Self-Treat Eye Problems

See your doctor promptly if any of the following are present:

1. Blurry or cloudy vision, particularly if the change is recent
2. Discharge of pus from the eye, with or without caking or sticking of the eyelids in the morning
3. Eye pain
4. A sore or ulcer in the eye
5. Anything more than a slight degree of redness
6. Severe itching
7. Redness beginning around the middle of the eye, rather than at the sides
8. Injury to the eye
9. Pale, itching eyes
10. Lumps or bumps on the eye or on the eyelid, particularly on the inside of the lids
11. Double vision
12. Blind spots or partial blindness of one or both eyes
13. Foreign bodies, if they persist

Eye Problems

Home Treatment

Home treatment may be initiated for the following symptoms:
1. Slight redness of one or both eyes
2. Mild dryness, burning, and discomfort
3. Mild degree of *clear* discharge
4. Mild itching

These symptoms usually indicate an allergy, a mild viral infection, lack of sleep, or an irritant such as smog, tobacco, fumes, wind, dust, or excessive sun. As emphasized above, it is easy to be fooled into believing that your problem is not serious, but remember, you are dealing with your vision.

There may be some degree of assurance that your eye symptoms are not due to serious disease when they occur in conjunction with a known cause, such as in association with the symptoms of a common cold. If you are sneezing and coughing and have a runny or stuffed nose, and if your eyes are somewhat red with a watery discharge, you can be fairly certain the eye problem is due to the same virus that is responsible for the cold. If you have allergies such as hay fever, and your eyes are dry, burning, and itchy during a hay-fever attack, it is likely that it is due to the same cause. If you have had an unusual degree of sun, wind, or fume exposure and your eyes are red, dry, and itchy, it is probably due to the environmental condition. However, when your eye condition occurs in isolation—without a known cause—and especially if the eye symptoms last more than two or three days, you should check with your doctor before continuing self-treatment. You must always keep in mind that redness of the eye, and other symptoms of trivial disease, may also be present when the difficulty is due to glaucoma, serious infection, tumors, etc.

Types of OTC Eye Preparations Available

1. *Cleansing agents.* Most of these preparations (Ocusol, etc.) contain a mild antiseptic, such as zepheran, which has cleansing properties. These products have never been shown to be more effective than splashing cool water in the eye, but they enjoy great popularity, nevertheless. Normal

tears contain far more antibacterial properties than most of the cleansing agents that are available OTC. In addition, these preparations occasionally act as irritants themselves, especially after prolonged usage. They are therefore best reserved for occasional use.

2. *Vasoconstrictors.* These agents act to narrow the diameter of blood vessels with which they come in contact. They are the same class of chemicals that are used in the common cold to shrink inflamed and swollen mucous membranes in the nose. When packaged for eye use, though, their concentration is considerably reduced.

Redness or "inflammation" of the eye is due to engorged and enlarged blood vessels in the conjunctiva. This is sometimes referred to as "pink eye." The vasoconstrictors will, on a temporary basis, constrict the blood vessels and thus reduce the redness and inflamed look of the eye. At times, adding a few drops of vasoconstrictor can be quite dramatic in changing the appearance of the eye. At one time—we hope the vogue has passed—it was quite fashionable for women to have "clear, white eyes," and they would use vasoconstrictors for cosmetic purposes. Some TV advertisements suggest the same use for these drugs. There is absolutely no medical reason to reduce the "bloodshot" appearance of eyes. When it is present for trivial reasons, it will usually disappear spontaneously in a day or so. If it does not, a physician should be consulted. If the eye feels dry, burning, and uncomfortable, cold compresses to the eye will usually give satisfactory relief.

In spite of this, eye products containing vasoconstrictors (with or without cleansing agents) are some of the most popular OTC products. The most commonly used vasoconstrictor is phenylephrine (Degest, Ocusol, etc.), but this chemical has its shortcomings; it decomposes rapidly in the bottle, and should not be used beyond three months after opening. It will, however, do an effective job in reducing "bloodshot" eyes for a few hours. Although tetrahydrozoline (Visine, Murine 2) is probably no more effective than preparations containing phenylephrine, it does have the advantage of being somewhat more stable than phenylephrine after opening, and is therefore preferred. Naphazoline (Allerest, Clear Eyes, Naphcon) is another effective vasoconstrictor.

3. *Artificial tears.* In addition to vasoconstrictors and cleansing agents, some preparations also contain "artificial tears." This compound is sometimes helpful in those conditions in which normal tears are reduced or insufficient. It is composed of a high-viscosity agent (thicker than water) that can substitute for normal tears when the latter are deficient or absent. Artificial tears sometimes are helpful with ordinary causes of dry, irritated, and smarting eyes, due to chemical irritants (smog, fumes, etc.), excessive sun exposure, and other physical and chemical agents. Some diseases are also characterized by reduced or absent tears (Sjögren's syndrome, etc.) There is very little difference between the various OTC products containing "artificial tears," and they may be chosen on the basis of personal preference and cost.

Suggested Treatment Plan for Minor Eye Irritations

1. Eliminate cause, such as tobacco smoke, excessive sun, etc., if possible.
2. Splash eyes with cool tapwater, as often as needed, or use cool compresses on the closed eyes.
3. For dry, irritated eyes without excessive redness, use artificial tears (any from group), two or three drops in each eye, as often as needed.
4. For inflamed eyes ("pink eye," "bloodshot eyes") accompanied by watery discharge, use a vasoconstrictor preparation such as Visine, two or three drops, two or three times a day. Do not continue for more than three days. If the problem persists, see your doctor.

If any of the symptoms listed on page 104 are present, do *not* self-treat; see your physician promptly.

Cleansing Agents ("Eye Washes")

Name	Approximate Cost
Blinx	1 oz. for $1.05
Collyrium	6 oz. for 1.61*
Eye-Stream	1 oz. for 1.54
Trisol Eye Wash	1 oz. for 1.59

* Best buy in group.

Vasoconstrictors

GROUP I
Recommended

Name	Approximate Cost
Albalon	½ oz. for $3.29†
Allerest	½ oz. for 1.79
Clear Eyes	½ oz. for 1.75†
Murine 2	½ oz. for 1.75
Naphcon	½ oz. for 3.15
Visine	½ oz. for 1.75

GROUP II
Acceptable

Examples of phenylephrine and other vasoconstrictor preparations

Name	Approximate Cost
Degest	½ oz. for $2.10
Eye Cool	¾ oz. for 2.00
Eyegenic Eye Mist/Drops	¼ oz. for 2.48
	½ oz. for 1.29
Isopto-Frin	½ oz. for 3.08†
Murine	½ oz. for 1.49
Ocusol Drops	½ oz. for 1.39†
Op-Isophrin	½ oz. for 1.75
Prefrin	½ oz. for 2.45†
Soothe	½ oz. for 1.75
Tear-efrin	½ oz. for 2.66†

Artificial Tears

Examples of artificial tears without vasoconstrictors

Name	Approximate Cost
Contique Artificial Tears	½ oz. for $2.59
Isopto Alkaline	½ oz. for 3.22
Isopto Plain	½ oz. for 2.59

† Also contains artificial tears.

Isopto Tears	½ oz. for	2.59
Lacril	½ oz. for	2.45
Liquifilm Tears	½ oz. for	2.45
Lyteers	½ oz. for	2.31
Tearisol	½ oz. for	2.45
Ultra Tears	½ oz. for	3.22

Chapter 12

Headaches

Not all headaches are the same, and not all headaches can be or should be treated with over-the-counter medication. It is important to recognize some of the various causes of headaches so that head pain due to serious disease, such as a brain tumor, can be brought to your doctor's attention as quickly as possible. There are also some types of headaches (migraine, for instance) which simply cannot be treated effectively with over-the-counter pain remedies. On the other hand, tension headaches, which are the most common form of headache, usually can be adequately handled with nonprescription pain medication.

Types of Headaches

1. Tension (muscle-contraction) headaches
2. Headaches associated with systemic illness, such as with flu, fever, and infections
3. Headaches due to fasting, eyestrain, hangover, and excessive sun
4. Headaches due to sinus infection
5. Migraine headaches
6. Headaches due to disease within the brain, such as brain tumor, stroke, meningitis, or encephalitis

Tension (Muscle-Contraction) Headaches

Almost every adult, and most children, have experienced a tension headache at one time or another. It is one of the most common symptoms to which man is prone. It also accounts for a large proportion of the over-the-counter drug market

Headaches

both in terms of available drugs and in terms of the amount of money spent on non-prescription preparations.

Tension headaches may occur at any age. They are usually associated with psychological stress and tension, or with physical fatigue. They may also develop for unknown reasons. The headache is generally felt in diffuse fashion over the entire head, but is sometimes more prominent in either the forehead or at the back of the head. It may be mild, and of nuisance value only, or quite severe. The discomfort is frequently described as "bandlike," or as an "aching sensation." Tension headaches may occur at any time of the day, but generally are worse as the day wears on. Some people notice the pain on arising in the morning, but the headaches almost never actually awaken the sufferer from a sound sleep, as do certain other forms of headache (see below).

Tension headaches are thought to be due to tension or muscular contraction of the posterior neck muscles (those at the back of the neck). Nerves going to the top and sides of the scalp pass through these muscles, and when the muscles go into "spasm," the nerves become irritated. This results in pain and discomfort in the region of the head which the nerves supply. This form of headache, then, is due to a temporary irritation of the nerves going to the scalp, and is not due to disease within the skull or brain.

Treatment of Tension Headaches

Since this is the most common form of headache, you have probably already had the experience of treating tension headaches with over-the-counter medication. Most of the widely advertised brands of pain relievers will reduce the head pain in 20 to 30 minutes after treatment is begun. However, this is not to imply that all brands are equally effective, equally safe, or of equal cost. Before describing the various preparations available, and their relative effectiveness, you should note the following points about the treatment of headaches in general.

1. Treat the symptom early. It requires less medication if the headache is treated soon after it begins, rather than later, when it may have intensified.
2. *All* drugs have side effects if taken too often and in exces-

sive amounts. Overtreatment may induce some of these side effects and compound your miseries.
3. You may have to experiment somewhat to see which of the available over-the-counter medicines is best suited to you, both in terms of relieving the head pain and in avoiding side effects.

Plain aspirin is the drug of choice for tension headaches. "Plain aspirin" means aspirin without additional ingredients such as extra painkillers, antacids, or stimulants.

For those people who cannot tolerate aspirin because of side effects such as stomach irritation, an alternate drug of choice is acetaminophen, which is contained in several over-the-counter products, including Tylenol, Tempra, etc. Acetaminophen has somewhat the same effectiveness for tension headaches as does aspirin but in some people it may have fewer side effects. It is, however, more costly than plain aspirin.

Most (but not all) of the widely advertised aspirin products contain more than just plain aspirin. The manufacturers claim that the additional ingredients result in "faster pain relief," or in "less irritation to the delicate lining of the stomach," or that their product is "stronger than plain aspirin," or contains "more of the pain reliever that doctors recommend most." The facts, however, rarely support the advertisers claims. For example:

1. *Combination drugs.* The addition of other drugs to a basic aspirin formula, such as in Anacin, Empirin, APC tablets etc., generally contributes nothing to the effectiveness of pain relief, but may contribute a good deal to the cost and to the possible side effects of the medication. Some combination formulas (such as those containing phenacetin) may even be dangerous.

Some of the formulas, such as Excedrin and Vanquish contain not only aspirin, but acetaminophen as well. This does not make much sense since the main advantage of acetaminophen is that it is tolerated by many persons susceptible to the side effects of aspirin. Combining them in a single drug destroys this advantage.

2. *Aspirin with antacids.* TV commercials have made us all aware of possible stomach upset with aspirin. The truth is that a small percentage of people who take aspirin will

indeed, experience some degree of stomach irritation. It is, however, quite unlikely that the tiny amount of antacid in Bufferin and similar preparations will do much in the way of preventing stomach distress. This effect can be minimized by taking aspirin with food or with a full glass of water. For those few people who cannot solve the problem in this way, no aspirin of any sort should be used, and a substitute should be tried (see below).

What about the speed of absorption of aspirin? Advertisers again make much of this property, showing graphs, charts, and diagrams of how one brand is absorbed into the blood stream more rapidly than another. It is indeed true that adding an antacid (yes, antacid!) to the formula (as in Bufferin, for instance) results in more rapid absorption of aspirin from the stomach into the blood stream. Dissolving the aspirin before it gets into the stomach and adding antacids as well (as in Alka-Seltzer) is even more efficient means of producing rapid absorption. However, the speed of absorption alone does not pass the "so-what test." The time difference between absorption of plain aspirin and buffered and/or dissolved aspirin is quite small, and from a practical point of view, it is not significant in terms of the time required to afford relief of pain.

3. *Other forms of aspirin.* Aspirin is available in chewing-gum form and in tablets which do not dissolve until they pass through the stomach into the intestine (enteric-coated tablets). Neither of these forms is recommended, since their absorption and effectiveness are not reliable. Time-release aspirins are likewise of little value in the treatment of tension headaches.

Recommended Dosage of Plain Aspirin (Adults)

Aspirin tablets come as 5 gr or 325 mg tablets. Both descriptions mean the same thing. Slight variations in the strength of the tablet, such as 300 mg or 350 mg, have no practical significance.

For occasional tension headaches, start with two tablets of plain aspirin. If they bother your stomach, take the tablets with food or with a full glass of water. If your headache is not relieved, take another two tablets in three hours. If your headache is still not significantly improved, take three more aspirin in four hours from the last dose. This may be repeated in four hours, if necessary. Do not take more than ten aspirin tablets in a 24-hour period without checking with your doctor. If you become nauseated or develop ringing in your ears, you have had too much aspirin and you should call your doctor before proceeding.

It is important not to take *any* amount of medicine on a day-in and day-out basis without it being specifically prescribed by your doctor. Even small amounts of aspirin, for instance, taken on a daily basis can produce side effects such as stomach bleeding with resulting anemia.

Acetaminophen

If aspirin cannot be tolerated because of side effects, it is best not to try to overcome these side effects with various aspirin combination formulas, but rather to go directly to acetaminophen medication such as Tylenol or Tempra. Tablet for tablet, acetaminophen has the same potency as aspirin, so the same treatment program can be used with this medication as has been described for aspirin.

Children's Dosage

Children can use plain aspirin for tension headaches. Children's aspirin (Bayer, St. Joseph) comes in 81-mg tablets. Approximately four children's tablets are equal to one adult aspirin tablet. One children's tablet can be given for every year of age, up to four or five years old. At that time, a single adult tablet can be used, dissolved or crushed in some jam or syrup, if your child cannot swallow the tablet whole. By age 10 or 12, two adult tablets can be used.

TREATMENT PLAN FOR TENSION HEADACHES (ADULTS)

Drug of Choice: Plain Aspirin
(325 mg or 5 gr)

Alternate Choice: acetaminophen

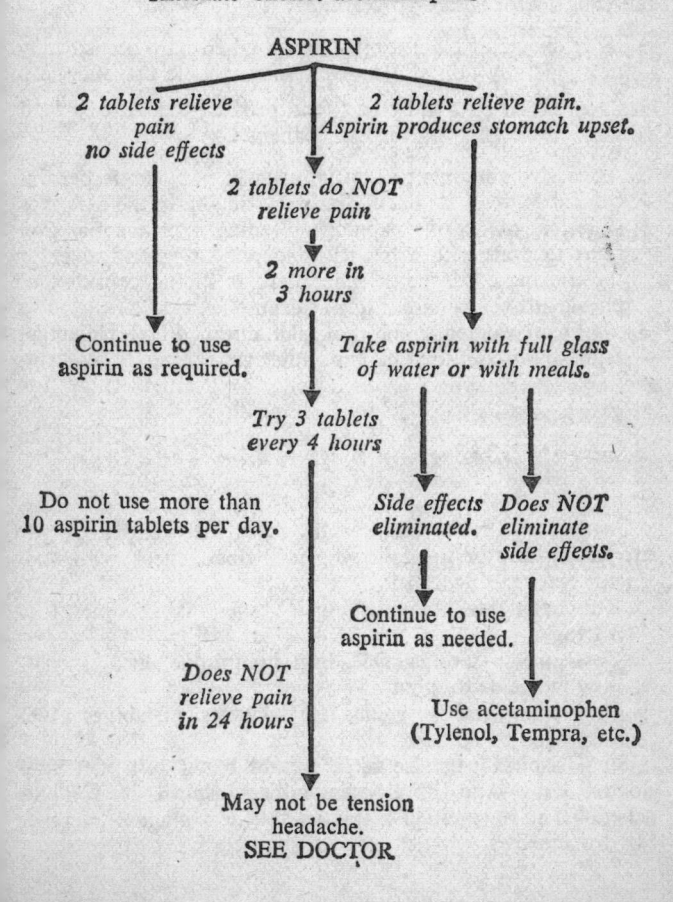

ASPIRIN

2 tablets relieve pain no side effects

2 tablets relieve pain. Aspirin produces stomach upset.

2 tablets do NOT relieve pain

2 more in 3 hours

Continue to use aspirin as required.

Take aspirin with full glass of water or with meals.

Try 3 tablets every 4 hours

Do not use more than 10 aspirin tablets per day.

Side effects eliminated.   *Does NOT eliminate side effects.*

Continue to use aspirin as needed.

Does NOT relieve pain in 24 hours

Use acetaminophen (Tylenol, Tempra, etc.)

May not be tension headache.
SEE DOCTOR

If liquid is preferred to tablets, it is best to use acetaminophen-containing medication (Tylenol, Tempra), which comes in both child and adult dosage forms. Follow the instructions on the label for correct dosage.

Side Effects of Aspirin

1. Side effects of plain aspirin, when taken only occasionally, are generally minor. However, some people are allergic to any dose of aspirin and may develop skin rash or asthma. If you are susceptible to allergies, do not take *any* aspirin without your doctor's approval.
2. Excessive amounts of aspirin, even in nonallergic persons, can cause upset stomach, dizziness, ringing in the ears, possible loss of hearing, stomach bleeding, and anemia. *Caution*: Persons with a history of peptic or gastric ulcer, or those using cortisone or other steroids should consult their physicians before taking *any* aspirin.
3. Pregnant women should not take *any* medicine (including aspirin) without their doctor's approval.

Aspirin's Interaction With Other Medicines

Aspirin can react with certain other medications. If you are taking any of the following medicines, check with your doctor before using aspirin:
1. Anticoagulants (blood thinners) such as Dicumerol or Warfarin
2. Cortisone or steroids (Decadron, prednisone, etc.)
3. Any medicine for gout
4. Oral hypoglycemic agents for diabetes (Diabinese, Orinase)

Since aspirin can also alter certain blood tests, let your doctor know you have been taking aspirin if you are scheduled to have either a thyroid test or a glucose-tolerance test for diabetes.

Special Note on Kidney Damage

It is believed by many physicians that prolonged use of phenacetin, a drug commonly employed in combination over-the-counter headache remedies (APC tablets, Bromo-Seltzer, Empirin, etc.), could lead to permanent kidney damage in some habitual users. Canada has banned its use except by prescription for this reason. In the United States, phenacetin-containing products must carry a warning not to take the drug "regularly for longer than 10 days without consulting your physician." Some investigators, however, believe the problem is not confined to phenacetin, and any of the over-the-counter pain medications taken over prolonged periods of time can cause kidney damage.

It is clear that over-the-counter medication, including plain aspirin, should not be taken on a daily basis without a physiican's supervision. However, since phenacetin has been especially implicated in the kidney problem, it is best to avoid it completely.

Headaches Associated With Systemic Illnesses

Systemic illnesses that may involve headache include flu, fever, infections, and high blood pressure.

This type of headache has the same characteristics as tension headaches in that it is usually felt diffusely over the entire head and is generally of mild intensity.

Plain aspirin is again the drug of choice for these headaches. It is more important, however, to get at the source of the headache and obtain effective treatment for the underlying condition.

Headaches Due to Fasting, Eyestrain, Hangover, and Excessive Sun

If a specific cause for the headache is known, such as not having eaten for a prolonged period, the obvious treatment is to correct the cause. With all these headaches, however, plain aspirin will help eliminate or reduce the immediate pain.

"Headaches" Due to Sinus Infection

These are, strictly speaking, not headaches at all. They are caused by infection or blockage of one or more of the sinuses about the face and head. They are usually associated with other symptoms of sinusitis such as fever and running or stuffy nose. They are sometimes associated with allergies. Although plain aspirin may give some temporary relief, your doctor should be consulted for more definitive treatment.

Migraine Headaches

This variety of headache is sometimes referred to as "sick headache" because it is frequently associated with nausea and vomiting. The pain is usally one-sided and may be throbbing, rather than steady, in nature. Visual disturbances such as blind spots, flashing lights, and halos may either precede or accompany the headache. Certain varieties of migraine can be associated with temporary neurological manifestations such as speech difficulty, limb weakness or numbness, or brief periods of actual blindness. Several members of a family may be affected.

Over-the-counter medications are usually *in*effective for the relief of this type of headache. However, if it is caught early, three aspirin may provide some benefit, though usually incomplete. Your doctor can prescribe medication which is designed to either prevent the headache from occurring, or control it once it has begun.

Headaches Due to Disease Within the Brain

Brain tumor, stroke, meningitis, encephalitis, and other brain diseases produce headaches.

Headaches

These headaches are usually, but not always, more severe than tension headaches and are generally more prolonged. The pain may be diffuse or it may be felt in a localized area of the head. It may awaken the patient from a sound sleep.

Although aspirin and other over-the-counter medication may temporarily relieve the head pain, should any of the symptoms listed below occur in association with a headache, let your doctor know promptly.

1. Severe nausea and vomiting
2. Visual difficulties, including double vision or blindness
3. Speech difficulty
4. Weakness, tingling, or numbness in the limbs
5. Walking difficulty
6. Incoordination
7. Alteration in your usual alertness
8. One-sided headache
9. The headache awakens you from a deep sleep
10. Stiff neck, with or without fever
11. Headache persists for more than a couple of days
12. Over-the-counter medication does not relieve the headache

Aspirin

GROUP I
Recommended

Examples of plain aspirin without additional ingredients

A. Adult aspirin

Name	Approximate Cost
Plain aspirin (various manufacturers and distributors —Whiteworth, Safeway, Thrifty, etc.)	100 tablets for $0.29*
Bayer Aspirin	100 tablets for 1.54
Stanco	12 tablets for 0.25
St. Joseph Aspirin	100 tablets for 0.89

* Best buy in group.

B. Children's aspirin

Name	Approximate Cost
Bayer Children's Aspirin (1¼ gr.)	36 tablets for 0.59
St. Joseph Aspirin for Children (1¼ gr.)	36 tablets for 0.59

GROUP II
Acceptable

Examples of aspirin preparations containing additional but unnecessary ingredients

Name	Additional Ingredients	Approximate Cost
Alka-Seltzer	Antacid	25 tablets for $1.03
Anacin	Caffeine	100 tablets for 1.97
Ascriptin	Antacid	100 tablets for 1.79
B.C. Powder	Caffeine, salicylamide	50 packets for 1.69
B.C. Tablets	Caffeine, salicylamide	100 tablets for 1.69
Buffered aspirin (various manufacturers and distributors)	Antacid	100 tablets for 0.80*
Bufferin	Antacid	100 tablets for 1.95
Fizrin	Antacid	24 tablets for 1.38
Stanback Powder	Caffeine, salicylamide	50 packets for 1.59
Stanback Tablets	Caffeine, salicylamide	100 tablets for 1.59

* Best buy in group.

GROUP III
Unacceptable

A. Examples of aspirin preparations containing potentially harmful ingredients

Name	Additional Ingredient
APC tablets & capsules	Phenacetin
ASA tablets & capsules	Phenacetin
Capron	Phenacetin
Congespirin	Decongestant
Cope	Antihistamine
Empirin Compound	Phenacetin
Excedrin P.M.	Antihistamine
4-Way Cold Tablet	Decongestant
Midol	Phenacetin
PAC	Phenacetin
Sine-Aid	Decongestant
Sine-Off	Antihistamine

B. Examples of aspirin preparations in nonrecommended form

Name	Form	Comment
ASA Enseals	Enteric-coated	Unreliable absorption
Aspergum	Chewing gum	Unreliable blood levels from gum
Bayer Timed Release Aspirin	Time release	No advantage for treatment of headaches
Measurin	Time release	No advantage for treatment of headaches

Acetaminophen

GROUP I
Recommended

Examples of plain acetaminophen

A. Adult acetaminophen

Name	Approximate Cost		
Acetaminophen (various manufacturers and distributors— Safeway, Thrifty, etc.)	100 tablets	for	$1.25*
Apamide	100 tablets	for	2.80
Bayer Non-Aspirin Pain Reliever	100 tablets	for	2.10
Datril	100 tablets	for	2.10
Fendon	100 tablets	for	1.61
Nebs	100 tablets	for	2.88
Proval	100 tablets	for	2.66
	100 capsules	for	12.95
	16 oz. elixir	for	6.93
SK-APAP	100 tablets	for	2.03
	4 oz. elixir	for	1.33
Tempra	100 tablets	for	4.06
Trilium	50 tablets	for	1.65
Tylenol	100 tablets	for	2.20
Tylenol Extra Strength (500 mg)	100 tablets	for	2.50
Valadol	100 tablets	for	2.59
Valgesic	12 packets	for	3.00

B. Children's acetaminophen

Name	Approximate Cost	
Proval drops	½ oz.	for 1.26
St. Joseph Fever Reducer for Children	½ oz. drops	for 1.19
	2 oz. elixir	for 0.99
Tempra drops	½ oz.	for 1.45
Tylenol drops	½ oz.	for 1.60

* Best buy in group.

GROUP II
Acceptable

Examples of acetaminophen preparations containing additional but unnecessary ingredients. Acetaminophen is best used in persons in whom aspirin is not well tolerated (stomach upset, rash, etc.). Combinations containing acetaminophen plus aspirin destroy the usefulness of acetaminophen for these persons. Group II is "acceptable" only because the ingredients are not generally harmful, but the preparations containing aspirin are not very rational and are not recommended.

Name	Additional Ingredients	Approximate Cost
Arthralgen	Salicylamide	100 tablets for $5.95
Excedrin	Aspirin, caffeine, salicylamide	100 tablets for 1.97*
Trigesic	Aspirin, caffeine	100 tablets for 2.65
Vanquish	Aspirin, caffeine antacids	100 tablets for 2.77

GROUP III
Unacceptable

Examples of acetaminophen preparations containing potentially harmful ingredients

Name	Additional Ingredient
Bromo Quinine Cold Tablets	Decongestant
Bromo-Seltzer	Phenacetin
Excedrin P.M.	Antihistamine
Percogesic	Antihistamine

---

* Best buy in group.

Chapter 13

Arthritis and Rheumatism, Neuralgia, Neuritis, and Muscle Aches and Pains

Arthritis and Rheumatism

To the average person, arthritis and rheumatism have similar meanings and these terms usually bring to mind a condition in which one or more joints of the body are diseased.

Commonly recognized symptoms include pain, stiffness and deformity of joints, and sometimes accompanying muscle aches and pains. These manifestations may vary from severe and acute pain, associated with swelling and redness of joints, to mild stiffness and aching of the joints, with all degrees of severity in between.

Technically, there is a difference between arthritis and rheumatism. Arthritis is a condition in which detectable inflammation of the joints occurs and is accompanied by pain, swelling, and redness. The term "rheumatism" is used by doctors to describe a condition in which the patient feels pain, aching, or stiffness in the joint(s) but no signs of inflammation can actually be detected. This does not imply that this condition is any less real or painful to the patient. Despite this technicality, these two terms are frequently used synonymously, and both of them occur in advertisements and day-to-day usage.

Joint complaints are extremely common. In the United States, well over 10 million people suffer from some form of rheumatism, and in England the percentage is much greater. It has been stated that over half the English population is afflicted with at least minor rheumatic troubles. It is no surprise that with this potential market, the OTC drug manufacturers have gone overboard. So, in fact, have pseudoscientists who have written books on the "cure" of arthritis by extraordinary means. One such popular work suggests that the joints be kept "greased" by diet. Arthritis is one of the areas of medicine (cancer is another) in which quacks, get-rich-quick artists, con men, and phony-device manufacturers abound—all to the detriment and expense of the victim of the disease.

Types of Arthritis

There are many types of arthritis, though only the most common forms will be discussed here. The three most common types of arthritis are listed below, and their similarities and differences are noted in the table on page 133.

1. Degenerative joint disease (osteoarthritis)
   A. Generalized (many joints of the body are involved)
   B. Localized (a single or a few joints of the body are involved)
      1) Due to trauma or injury to the joint
      2) Due to faulty posture
2. Rheumatoid arthritis
3. Gouty arthritis

Degenerative Joint Disease (Osteoarthritis)

Sometimes called "osteo," this is by far the most common form of arthritis. On the basis of X-ray examination, it is present in almost everyone over the age of 40, and may occur earlier in life. However, even though there may be evidence of osteo on X-ray, it does not mean that everyone has symptoms. Most people do not have trouble until their 50s and 60s, when it becomes very common to have a "touch of arthritis."

There are two major forms of osteoarthritis. *Localized* osteo is due to an injury to a joint such as an athletic injury, or an accident. This may result in arthritis of the injured joint years after the trauma. Certain occupations and activities lead to osteoarthritis. "Housemaid's knee," "tennis elbow," "carpenter's wrist," etc. are names which aptly describe the joint which is involved, as well as the cause of the condition. It is clear that repeated use and abuse of a joint is likely to result in eventual osteoarthritis of that joint.

The *generalized* form of osteoarthritis occurs without specific injury or abuse to any one joint. Many joints are likely to be involved. The joints of the hands, hips, knees, and spine are most often affected. In a sense, this form of osteo is also due to trauma of the joints, but in this case it is due to the normal wear and tear of the body as it ages. It is normal in the sense that almost everyone is affected. The constant daily use and motion of our joints produces over the years a certain amount of injury to the cartilage within the joints. The joint responds by the production of new bone in the area. New growth of bone in injured areas can be very helpful, such as occurs in the healing process of fractures. However, within joints the new production of bone is, in large measure, responsible for the discomfort and deformity of the joint. It is the injury to joint cartilage and a reactive new growth of bone that is responsible for the symptoms of osteoarthritis, whether it be the localized or generalized form.

Symptoms of Osteoarthritis

Pain is the major symptom. It begins quite gradually, usually over a period of years. The pain is usually mild and appears after use of the joint, subsiding with rest. Stiffness of the affected joints is common and is usually noticed after prolonged rest of the joint, as may occur after a night's sleep. The stiffness disappears in a few moments once the joint is used.

There may be some deformity of the joints, especially those of the fingers. Deformities, usually as bumps, are most commonly present in the joints closest to the tips of the fingers (Heberden's nodes). These bumps are due to the new growth of bone within the joint, and may be somewhat tender to the touch. This deformity may interfere with movement of the hand. These nodes are much more common in women, and there is a strong hereditary predisposition to their development.

Nodes may also appear in the middle joint of the fingers, but in osteo, these are much less common. Nodes in this location can sometimes be confused with the deformities of rheumatoid arthritis, which may occur in the same location. These are distinguishable in that in osteo, they are less painful, are not red or swollen, and are not associated with the other features of rheumatoid arthritis.

In addition to the joints of the hand, the knee, hip, and spine are frequently affected by osteoarthritis. When the hip is involved, walking becomes difficult and pain in the groin, the inside of the thigh, and sometimes the knee is noted with walking or weight-bearing. When the knee is involved, there is pain with walking, and frequently crepitation (a scraping feeling) is experienced.

Osteoarthritis of the spine is very common after middle age. It occurs primarily in the bones of the neck and the low back. Pain on motion, stiffness, and sometimes neurological signs such as tingling in the limbs, weakness of the muscles of the limbs, and severe radiating pain into the arms or legs can occur in this condition.

Features of Osteoarthritis—Summary

1. Single joint involvement may follow injury at any age.
2. Generalized osteo usually begins over the age of 50.
3. Onset is slow and insidious.
4. Pain is generally mild and is worse with joint motion. Rest affords relief.
5. Prolonged rest, however, may produce stiffness of joints, which is quickly relieved with resumption of joint motion.
6. Joints of the hands, knees, hips, and spine are most frequently affected.
7. Deformity of the finger joints is much more common in women and is hereditary.
8. There are no associated systemic problems such as fever, weight loss, or generalized weakness.

Treatment of Osteoarthritis

1. No medicine will cure or retard the process.
2. Aspirin is the drug of choice for the pain of osteo. Two or three aspirin—aspirin without additional ingredients—three or four times a day is best. The aspirin should be taken with a full glass of water or with meals. Do not use aspirin if you have a history of gastric or peptic ulcer, or if you are taking any other medication on a regular basis, unless

you first check with your doctor. Common side effects of aspirin are ringing in the ears and dizziness. If these occur, cut back on the dosage.

If aspirin results in stomach distress, even though taken with water or meals, an antacid such as Maalox or Gelusil (preferably liquid, but tablets are OK) taken with aspirin is much better than "buffered" aspirin such as Bufferin. It is also less expensive.

3. Weight reduction is advisable if overweight. This is very important since the additional weight the joints must support adds to the intensity of joint wear and tear.
4. Change of occupation may be necessary, depending on which joints are involved and what kind of work you do.
5. Rest of the involved joint(s) will afford temporary relief.
6. Either moist or dry heat may also be of some help.

Rheumatoid Arthritis

Unlike osteoarthritis, rheumatoid arthritis is not limited to joints only. In fact, most persons who develop rheumatoid arthritis first notice loss of appetite, weight loss, weakness, and increasing fatigue. Low-grade fever may be present. It is only several weeks later that aching and pain in the muscles and joints are noted.

Rheumatoid arthritis is more common in women than men and it is characteristic that the first attack occurs in the 30s, although it may begin at almost any age, including childhood. The joints of the hands, knees, and feet are generally the first to be involved. They eventually become swollen, painful, red, and hot. The joints are usually affected equally on both sides of the body, although the process may begin in just one joint, soon to be joined by its counterpart on the other side.

Other evidence of a generalized disease may also occur. Skin rash on the face or elsewhere, lumps under the skin (especially over pressure points, such as elbows), eye problems, muscle wasting, and even heart and kidney involvement can occur.

One of the characteristic symptoms of rheumatoid arthritis, unlike osteoarthritis, is the "jelling" phenomenon. This is the feeling of stiffness and difficulty in movement which occurs after a prolonged rest, such as upon wakening in the morning. With use of joints, the stiffness gradually disappears or is improved, with resulting increased ability to use the joint. There may be some stiffness after a prolonged rest in osteoarthritis as well, but this is relieved in just a few moments after use of the joint. In contrast, the "jelling" phenomenon or stiffness of the joints in rheumatoid arthritis is not relieved for several hours after first use of the joints. A mild degree of exercise generally improves the symptoms of rheumatoid arthritis, in contrast to osteoarthritis, in which exercise increases the symptoms. Overdoing the exercise will make even rheumatoid arthritis worse.

The symptoms of rheumatoid arthritis come and go. There are frequently periods—of varying lengths—where all or most of the symptoms spontaneously disappear. Unfortunately, in most victims of this disease, they will reappear. However, in 10 to 20 percent of patients with rheumatoid arthritis, the symptoms do not recur. This may happen at almost any stage of the disease, so there is always hope for these sufferers. Disabilities and deformities that may already be present will not revert to normal, but at least there is a chance that the disease will not progress.

Features of Rheumatoid Arthritis—Summary

1. It is more common in women than men.
2. It usually begins in the 30s.
3. It is associated with loss of appetite, weight loss, fatigue, and fever.
4. It may be associated with other manifestations such as skin, muscle, heart, eye, and internal-organ involvement.
5. Stiffness and pain are worse in the morning, but improve with moderate exercise.
6. Symptoms are intermittent and there is a chance of a spontaneous remission.
7. For most victims, the disease is progressive over many years and serious deformities may eventually result.

Treatment of Rheumatoid Arthritis

It is essential that treatment of this condition be initiated and supervised by your physician. Although aspirin therapy is the cornerstone of treatment, there are many other drugs which are available only by prescription and which are beneficial for this condition.

When aspirin is prescribed by your physician, it will probably be in high doses, such as three or four tablets anywhere from four to six times a day. Plain aspirin—aspirin without additional components or drugs—should be used. A full glass of water with each dose, or aspirin taken with meals, will help prevent stomach irritation. If this is still a problem, an ounce of antacid such as Maalox or Gelusil should be used along with the aspirin. Antacids are much better and cheaper than using buffered aspirin such as Bufferin.

Aspirin should not be used without your doctor's approval if you are taking anticoagulants (blood thinners) or any other medication on a regular basis. The most frequent side effects of aspirin are ringing in the ears, dizziness, and stomach distress. Most patients with rheumatoid arthritis tolerate large doses of aspirin quite well, especially if the dosage is built up over a period of a few weeks. However, notify your doctor if ringing in the ears develops. He will probably reduce your dosage, but if there is a recurrent attack of the arthritis, he may have to add other drugs.

1. Acetaminophen preparations such as Tylenol and Tempra, although relatively effective painkillers (almost as good as aspirin), are not as good for arthritis as is plain aspirin. In rheumatoid arthritis, aspirin has a definite anti-inflammatory effect which works to reduce the inflammation of the arthritis as well as to relieve its pain. Tylenol and the other acetaminophen preparations do no more than relieve pain.
2. Rest is very important in the treatment of rheumatoid arthritis. Most physicians feel that several hours of bed rest each day are quite beneficial.
3. Graded exercises and physical therapy can be very helpful, and these should be initiated under the guidance of your physician, or of a physical therapist to whom your physician may send you.
4. A normal, well-balanced diet is all that is required. There are no diets that are going to "grease" your joints or otherwise improve rheumatoid arthritis.
5. The less weight your joints must carry, the better off they will be. Weight reduction is a *must* for overweight patients with this disease.
6. Application of heat, and sometimes cold, may offer considerable symptomatic relief.

7. Liniments and lotions irritate the skin, thus bringing blood to the surface and increasing the temperature in this location. This can afford some minor and temporary relief but it is not a good idea to use this form of treatment over a prolonged period of time. Some of the chemicals in these liniments are absorbed into the blood stream, so they are best reserved for occasional use. A heating pad is more efficient, cheaper, and less messy in providing heat to an area. *Do not use liniments and heating pads at the same time. Burns may result.*

Gout

Thomas Sydenham, a famous physician of his day and a gout sufferer, wrote in 1683, presumably from firsthand knowledge, ". . . the gout generally attacks those aged persons who have spent most of their lives in ease, voluptuousness, high living, and too free use of wine and other spiritous liquors." Although amusing to us today, there is no real evidence that "high living" has much to do with the disease. It is true that many famous and highly accomplished persons have been afflicted with gout. Isaac Newton, Martin Luther, John Calvin, Leonardo da Vinci, and Benjamin Franklin are just a few of the many notables who have had gout. But can we not say the same thing about other diseases: Heart disease, cancer, and strokes have also affected many famous, as well as ordinary, people throughout history. But the symptoms of gout are so dramatic that when they occur they are inescapable to the sufferer and all those around him.

Although there are other forms and possible complications of gout, arthritis is the symptom which usually heralds the disease. This takes the form of *extremely* painful swelling of the joint, usually associated with redness, heat, tenderness, and inability to move the involved joint. Fever and a generalized ill feeling may accompany the arthritis. The big toe is the area usually affected, but gout may also occur in the ankle, instep, knee, elbow, or wrist. The joint pain occasionally follows some trauma, such as an accident, a long walk, exposure to cold, or even psychological "trauma."

Before pain develops, there may be a feeling of burning, tingling, or aching in the joint, soon followed by the arthritis.

As often as not, though, it begins *very* quickly—within a few minutes to perhaps a few hours—with the development of severe pain, swelling, redness, and heat in the joint. It may even begin in the middle of the night. When untreated, the inflammation lasts a week or two and then spontaneously subsides. About two-thirds of all those with an attack of gout will have a subsequent attack within the first year. Between 5 and 10 percent of affected persons will have only a single attack in their lives. There are usually no symptoms of arthritis between these acute attacks, unless the disease becomes chronic.

Gout is a male disease; women are only rarely affected, and then usually only after menopause. It is a familial disease, and so it is more likely to occur within families than sporadically in the general population. But even in afflicted families there is only a 10 to 20 percent chance of direct heredity.

It is important to realize that gout, in addition to the dramatic arthritis which occurs, is a disease that may have significant complications in other organs of the body, especially the kidneys. Gout on occasion is associated with other diseases, such as diabetes and psoriasis. It is especially important, therefore, to seek medical advice when an attack of gout occurs.

Features of Gout—Summary

1. It cannot be cured.
2. There is excellent medication (which only a physician can prescribe) which can control the acute attacks of gout and help prevent any possible complications of the disease.
3. Gout may be associated with other diseases—another good reason to be checked by your doctor.
4. Chronic gouty arthritis can frequently be prevented by appropriate prescription medication.
5. *There is no OTC medication which is effective for gout. Do not try to self-treat, even if the first attack subsides by itself.*

Types of Arthritis

Type/Characteristics	Generalized Osteoarthritis	Rheumatoid Arthritis	Gout
USUAL AGE OF OCCURRENCE	OVER 40	UNDER 40	OVER 40
Sex preponderance	Females more than males	Females more than males	Mostly men, occasionally females after menopause
Onset	Over years	Over weeks	Rapid; minutes to hours
Is there swelling or tenderness of joints?	Mild to moderate	Definite	Definite
Is there deformity of joints?	Mild	Yes	Yes, if disease becomes chronic; especially in the big toe
Which joints are usually involved?	Hands, hips, knees, spine	Hands, knees, feet	Big toe, ankle, instep, knee, elbow, wrist
Is there fever, rash, sick feeling present?	No	Yes	Occasionally
Are there recurrent attacks?	No, symptoms are steady	Yes	Yes
Is stiffness worse in the morning?	Slightly	Yes ("jelling phenomenon")	No
What's the effect of exercise?	Worsened with exercise	Stiffness is improved with *mild* exercise	Worsened by any joint movement

Neuralgia and Neuritis

Neuralgia is a term used to indicate a disturbance of the peripheral nerves of the arms, legs, and sometimes the chest. Neuritis is used synonymously by most people, but it occasionally has the added connotation of a more acute or more severe condition.

Nerves innervate all the muscles of the body, the skin, and most of the internal organs. *Motor nerves* carry the electrical "messages" *from* the brain and spinal cord which direct muscular and organ activity. *Sensory nerves* carry messages *to* the spinal cord and brain, conveying sensations of pain, heat and cold, limb position, texture, and other sensory information.

When these nerves are disturbed by disease, one of two things (or a combination of the two) can occur: (1) If motor nerves are affected, there may be weakness and/or incoordination of the muscles. (2) When the sensory nerves are affected, there will be difficulty with the perception of touch, pain, and other sensations. There may also be spontaneous sensory sensations such as numbness, tingling, pins-and-needle sensations, and burning feelings. These spontaneous sensations are what is generally referred to as neuralgia or neuritis.

There is a long list of causes of neuraligia and neuritis. Striking the "funny bone" of the elbow is an example of an acute form of neuritis. It is caused by a minor injury to a nerve in the elbow. Pins and needles in the leg and foot, due to compression of nerves in the knee by prolonged sitting with knees crossed, is another example. Some of the more serious conditions that can lead to chronic neuritis and neuralgia are:

1. Severe injury to a nerve
2. Diabetes, which sometimes results in difficulty in walking and sensory disturbances
3. Toxins, such as lead poisoning, which may result in weakness of the hand and other muscles
4. Infectious diseases, such as certain viruses, which can produce weakness and sensory disturbances in the limbs
5. Hereditary problems, where abnormalities in peripheral nerves occur in families
6. Vitamin deficiencies, such as vitamin B-12 abnormalities resulting in pernicious anemia

Arthritis and Rheumatism

7. Chronic alcoholism, which may lead to Vitamin B-1 deficiency, with resulting difficulty in walking and sensory abnormalities

If the symptoms of neuraligia and neuritis, such as tingling, numbness, pins-and-needles sensations, etc., persist for more than a few days, they should certainly be checked by your doctor, since they may indicate an underlying condition which requires medical attention.

Muscle Aches and Pains

Muscle aching is most frequently due to strain on the muscle by unaccustomed exercise. Occasionally it is due to inflammation of the muscles or a reaction to internal abnormalities. As in neuralgia, if muscle aching with no obvious explanation persists for more than a few days, a physician should be consulted.

Suggested Treatment of Neuritis, Neuralgia, and Muscle Aches and Pains

1. Rest the affected part of the body.
2. Apply heat, either moist or dry.
3. Take plain aspirin in doses of two or three tablets, three or four times a day. All the precautions outlined in Chapter 12 should be observed when using large amounts of aspirin. If aspirin cannot be tolerated because of stomach distress, ringing in the ears, or dizziness, acetaminophen preparations such as Tylenol, SK-APAP, Nebs, etc. may be substituted for aspirin. Take in the same dosage as aspirin (two or three tablets, three or four times a day). *Note*: Acetaminophen preparations are useful for the relief of pain *only*, and *do not* affect the inflammatory reaction of arthritis.
4. Liniments and lotions are sometimes useful on a temporary basis, but have little to offer over other methods of heat application. See pages 129-130 on treatment of rheumatoid arthritis for details.

When to See the Doctor

1. Any arthritis or rheumatism, muscle aches, or neuralgia lasting more than a week or so
2. Any arthritis associated with fever, sick feelings, eye trouble, rash, or shortness of breath
3. Any arthritis associated with swelling, pain, redness of joints
4. Recurrent attacks of any form of arthritis or muscle pains
5. Radiating pain in legs or arms, whether severe or mild
6. Wasting of limb muscles
7. If symptoms are not relieved by aspirin, rest, or heat
8. Any reaction to or difficulty in taking aspirin

Oral Medications for Arthritis and Rheumatism, Neuritis, Neuralgia, and Muscle Aches and Pains

Note: Acetaminophen is not as specific for arthritis as aspirin and is effective only in relief of pain. Aspirin will also help reduce inflammation.

GROUP I
Recommended

Plain aspirin—2 or 3 tablets, 3 or 4 times a day, with a full glass of water or with meals

GROUP II
Acceptable

Acetaminophen (Tylenol, Datril, Nebs, etc.)—2 or 3 tablets, 3 or 4 times a day

Externally Applied OTC Medication for Arthritis and Rheumatism, Neuritis, Neuralgia, and Muscle Aches and Pains

These products include liniments (ointment-like preparations) and lotions (liquid preparations). They are applied externally to the skin of the involved area and result in a feeling of warmth and comfort. They work mainly by producing a mild irritation in the skin, thus increasing the blood flow to that area. They may also work by directly interfering with pain fibers within the skin, thus alleviating some of the discomfort.

This group of medication is known as counterirritants. The most popular, and probably the most effective, medicine within this group is methyl salicylate. Chemically, methyl salicylate is related to aspirin. It is one of the few medicines that can pass through the skin barrier and get into the blood stream by vigorous rubbing onto the skin. Although it does not ordinarily produce its beneficial effect in this manner, continuous use over a prolonged period of time may produce a measurable amount of aspirinlike products in the blood stream. Liniments and lotions containing methyl salicylate therefore should not be used on a daily and long-term basis.

Another note of caution about methyl salicylate: It has been one of the major causes of accidental poisoning in children. One teaspoonful of methyl salicylate is equivalent to about 12 adult aspirin! Several years ago the Federal Food and Drug Administration required that products containing more than 5 percent methyl salicylate must be marketed in child-resistant containers and carry a warning to "Keep Out of Reach of Children."

Other drugs such as menthol, camphor, thymol, and clove oil are also used for their counterirritating effect. Most external OTC preparations for arthritis contain a combination of these products, with or without methyl salicylate.

The list in Group I cites examples of some of the OTC preparations available. All those chosen contain methyl salicylate, but other ingredients are usually present. There does not appear to be a significant medical difference between these preparations. The choice between liniment and lotion is strictly one of personal preference.

The preparations in Group II contain a local anesthetic. Local anesthetics cannot penetrate intact skin and may cause troubles of their own. Preparations containing this drug, therefore, are not recommended.

Liniments and Lotions

GROUP I
Acceptable

A. Examples of liniments (ointmentlike preparations). All preparations listed are of approximately equal benefit.

Name	Approximate Cost
Analgebalm	2 oz. for $1.34
Arthralgen	1 oz. for 1.58
Ben-Gay	1¼ oz. for 1.39
Deep Strength	1¼ oz. for 1.45
Mentholatum Deep Heating Rub	1¼ oz. for 1.29
Minit-Rub	1½ oz. for 1.15
SPD Analgesic Cream	1½ oz. for 0.84

B. Examples of lotions (liquid preparations). All preparations listed below are of approximately equal benefit.

Name	Approximate Cost
Analbalm	4 oz. for $1.82
Ben-Gay Lotion	2 oz. for 1.49
Heet	2⅓ oz. for 1.55
Mentholatum Deep Heating Lotion	2 oz. for 1.39
Panalgesic	4 oz. for 2.10
Sloan's Liniment	2 oz. for .89*
SPD Liquid	4 oz. for 1.33

GROUP II
Not Recommended

The following contain local anesthetic.

Exocaine
Exocaine Plus

---

* Best buy in group.

Chapter 14

Overweight Problems

Americans are notorious for eating too much and exercising too little. The result is that about 40 percent of the adult population is overweight. How do you know when you are overweight? Most of the time it is patently obvious, and if your best friends won't tell you, your mirror will. For those who wish to be scientific about it, the table on page 140 indicates desirable weights for American adults. If you exceed the upper weight in your category, you are overweight. If you are 20 pounds or more in excess of your ideal weight, you are obese.

For once, most physicians can agree with TV commercials—fat is *not* beautiful (medically, neither is skinny). Manufacturers of OTC weight-reduction medication resort to the physical appearance of fatness to make their pitch. They miss the point. Overweight is undesirable because it is associated with a shorter life span, as well as many medical problems (plus some psychological ones) while you are still around. Some of the diseases associated with excess weight are:

1. Atherosclerosis (hardening of the arteries) and resulting heart and kidney troubles
2. High blood pressure
3. Diabetes
4. Gallstones and gallbladder disease
5. Arthritis
6. Varicose veins

This does not imply that being overweight will necessarily cause all these problems or shorten one's life. Rather, being overweight is statistically associated with a high incidence of these illnesses. Even relatively small amounts of excess weight put you in a high-risk category for these diseases, as well as in a lower longevity category.

Desirable Weights for Men
and Women According to Height and
Frame, Ages 25 and Over[a]

	Weight in pounds (in indoor clothing)		
Height (in shoes)[b]	Small frame	Medium frame	Large frame
Men			
5 ft 2 in	112-120	118-129	126-141
5 ft 3 in	115-123	121-133	129-144
5 ft 4 in	118-126	124-136	132-148
5 ft 5 in	121-129	127-139	135-152
5 ft 6 in	124-133	130-143	138-156
5 ft 7 in	128-137	134-147	142-161
5 ft 8 in	132-141	138-152	147-166
5 ft 9 in	136-145	142-156	151-170
5 ft 10 in	140-150	146-160	155-174
5 ft 11 in	144-154	150-165	159-179
6 ft 0 in	148-158	154-170	164-184
6 ft 1 in	152-162	158-175	168-189
6 ft 2 in	156-167	162-180	173-194
6 ft 3 in	160-171	167-185	177-199
6 ft 4 in	164-175	172-190	182-204
Women			
4 ft 10 in	92-98	96-107	104-119
4 ft 11 in	94-101	98-110	106-122
5 ft 0 in	96-104	101-113	109-124
5 ft 1 in	99-107	104-116	112-128
5 ft 2 in	102-110	107-119	115-131
5 ft 3 in	105-113	110-122	118-134
5 ft 4 in	108-116	113-126	121-138
5 ft 5 in	111-119	116-130	125-142
5 ft 6 in	114-123	120-135	129-146
5 ft 7 in	118-127	124-139	133-150
5 ft 8 in	122-131	128-143	137-154
5 ft 9 in	126-135	132-147	141-158
5 ft 10 in	130-140	136-151	145-163
5 ft 11 in	134-144	140-155	149-168
6 ft 0 in	138-148	144-159	153-174

[a]Prepared by the Metropolitan Life Insurance Company. Derived primarily from data of the Build and Blood Pressure Study, 1959.
[b]Based on 1-inch heels for men and 2-inch heels for women.

How Does Overweight Develop?

1. *Eating.* In an otherwise healthy person, the "equation" for the *maintenance* of body weight is "input=output." "Input" is the number of calories we ingest by way of food and drink. "Output" is the number of calories we utilize as a result of normal body mechanisms (such as breathing, heartbeat, etc.), plus the physical exercise we do. An average male, between 20 and 40 years of age, utilizes about 3,000 calories per day; an average female, about 2,200. As long as input is equal to output (eating *and* utilizing 3,000 calories per day for males, 2,200 for females), there will be neither loss nor gain of body weight. We lose weight when output is in excess of input, and gain weight when we take in more calories than we expend. In other words, if more calories are consumed than are used, weight gain will result.

For instance, if you ate normally and used no energy (which, of course, is impossible—although some of us try hard to reach this "ideal"), you would gain about a pound a day. On the other hand, if you carried on normal activities and fasted, you would lose about a pound a day. If you ate twice as much in one day as you normally do, you would also gain a pound, assuming normal activity. It is not hard to see, therefore, how easy it is to gain weight. Over the course of a month, for example, if you ate just one "extra" day's worth of food (only about 3,000 calories), you would gain a pound a month, 12 pounds a year. If you kept this up for a couple of years you would be obese.

What happens to calories which are eaten and are not used up? Generally, the calories are converted to fat and deposited in fat cells. It has recently been shown that overeating in young children results in a greater number of fat cells, whereas overeating in adults results in greater deposition of fat in already existing fat cells. Because it is easier to remove fat from existing cells (by converting it back into calories and energy) than it is to reduce the number of fat cells, obesity in children is a more difficult problem to treat and carries a high probability of continuing into adulthood.

2. *Other factors contributing to weight gain.* Obesity has a tendency to run in families. In addition to the family environment, which may influence the person to overeat, there is probably a true genetic basis for obesity.

Certain medical diseases, such as endocrine abnormalities, are a rare cause of overweight. Underactive thyroid and other physical reasons for obesity have been much exaggerated. It is clear that at least 90 percent of all overweight persons in the United States eat excessive amounts (in relation to their needs) for psychological, cultural, and environmental reasons. In addition, habit plays a part, as do other mechanisms such as the aging process. It will no doubt seem strange, but the body is more efficient in its utilization of food as it ages, and therefore requires fewer calories. It is very common for the elderly to gain weight because their requirement for food decreases as a consequence both of increased efficiency of the utilization of food and of reduced activity (which also results in a lesser need for food). Eating the same number of calories when you get older as you did when you were younger will result in weight gain.

3. *Exercise.* The "output" side of the weight-maintenance equation consists of two parts: the calories utilized by internal bodily functions, such as breathing, heartbeat, etc., and the calories utilized by physical activity.

We obviously do not have much control over breathing and other internal bodily functions, so the most important means available to us for influencing the "output" side of the equation is through physical exercise. Unfortunately, it takes an awful lot of exercise to utilize the food we have eaten. For instance, bicycle riding at a normal speed uses only 200 calories an hour (equivalent to the caloric content of one scoop of chocolate ice cream). Tennis will result in a loss of 425 calories for each hour played (equivalent to the caloric content of one cheese sandwich). Walking at 2 miles per hour uses only 168 calories per hour (equivalent to one chocolate bar or one martini). It is not until very vigorous exercise occurs, such as swimming the backstroke (almost 2,000 calories per hour), that exercise alone can make a significant difference in the "input-output" equation.

It would therefore seem much easier to refrain from eating excessively if you wish to lose weight than to try to expend the extra calories by vigorous exercise, and this is perfectly true. However, the benefits of exercise go beyond the mere utilization of calories. In the first place, exercise tones up the body and gives one a sense of well-being. More important, from the standpoint of weight reduction, exercise seems to *reduce* appetite, and appetite is a major controller of how much we eat. On the other hand, decreased physical activity increases appetite!

Summary

1. Weight *maintenance* depends on ingesting the same number of calories as are used.
2. Weight *gain* occurs when more calories are ingested than are used.
3. Weight *loss* occurs when fewer calories are ingested than are used.
4. Exercise helps to utilize calories, but more important, it decreases appetite.

Treatment of Mild to Moderate Overweight Problems

In theory, losing weight is simple: Take in fewer calories than are used. In practice, this is like trying to stop a temper tantrum by spanking. The essential (and perhaps only) ingredient needed to lose weight is motivation. (What would we give for a "motivation pill"?) The motivation must be strong enough to withstand hunger pangs, the sights and sounds of eating, memories of food delights, boredom, habit, psychological instincts, social pressures to eat and drink, etc. To believe food faddists who claim that one can overcome all these lifelong reasons *not* to diet by some simplistic scheme is simply foolish. There is no such thing as a "simple" diet, a "simple" pill to lose weight, a "simple" exercise plan, or a "simple" anything, when it comes to weight reduction. Do not kid yourself about it. It is painfully hard work to lose weight, and you must want very badly to do so to be successful.

Severely overweight persons have essentially no chance of losing significant amounts of weight on their own and should begin their reduction program under the direction of a competent physician. On the other hand, for mildly or moderately overweight persons, it is not too difficult to lose a few pounds with almost any diet, since at first, most of the weight loss is due to loss of water. It is another matter to maintain the weight loss. Very few people are sufficiently motivated to put up with the difficulty and displeasure of chronic dieting. Only a small number of dieters can claim a weight loss after a few months or a year of "trying."

When dieting is begun, after the initial loss of "free" water, the first tissue to be reduced is protein, not fat. Protein contains a much higher concentration of water than fat does (about ten times as much), so that protein is much heavier on a volume-for-volume basis than fat. This accounts for much of the early weight loss. With continued dieting, however, the protein loss stabilizes and fat will then be lost. This is a much slower process, so it appears to the dieter that his weight has reached a "plateau" after only a few pounds of reduction. This is often so discouraging that the diet is abandoned and there is a return to the usual eating habits with resultant increase in weight. On the other hand, if the reason for this plateau is understood and dieting is continued, there will be a reduction in weight as a result of fat loss (as long as fewer calories are ingested than are used).

A reasonable goal of dieting is to aim to lose a pound a week, after the initial rapid loss. This can be accomplished by eating a diet which is only 500 calories per day less than the calories you use. This is equivalent to the caloric content of a single hamburger on a bun. If an increased amount of exercise is added, so much the better. As noted, exercise will help reduce appetite.

Aids to Dieting

1. *Diet pills.* There is no medication available, either by prescription or OTC, that reduces appetite without producing unwanted side effects. The diet pills prescribed by doctors are mostly derivatives of amphetamine (Benzedrine, Dexedrine, "uppers," "bennies"). These give the user a

Overweight Problems

sense of well-being and frequently reduce the desire to eat. They can sometimes be helpful at the beginning of dieting when some patients find it difficult to get started. They are *not* effective without a simultaneous reducing program. Furthermore, their effect usually wears off in a few weeks and then a letdown feeling, and sometimes depression, may occur. Amphetamines are also subject to abuse, and in the past few years this class of medicine has been closely regulated by the Food and Drug Administration. In spite of this, some physicians find these pills a useful adjunct in initiating the weight reduction process.

2. *Thyroid and other hormones*. Another popular medication used for dieting purposes is thyroid extract or its equivalent. In the *unusual* case of obesity due to underactive thyroid function, the use of replacement thyroid hormone is very specific and may be all that is needed to place the patient in hormonal balance and return him to normal weight. However, if thyroid disease is not present, the use of thyroid medication will not help in weight reduction. Furthermore, there are recent (1976) reports of an increased incidence of breast cancer in women who have used thyroid medication on a long-term basis, when thyroid disease was not present.

Several other hormones (other than thyroid) have been tried for weight-reduction purposes, and although they are still in the experimental stages, the results are not very encouraging for general use.

3. *Miscellaneous drugs*. A wide variety of medications and concoctions have been advocated at one time or another as a cureall for overweight. None have proved effective and some are harmful.

4. *Canned diet foods*. The first canned diet to gain popularity was Metrecal. There have since been several competitors (Sego, Slender, etc.). If used as directed, they all feature a 900-calorie-a-day diet. Since most adults utilize more than 900 calories a day, this diet will almost always result in weight loss. Furthermore, the makeup of the diet is reasonably well balanced, although certain minerals and vitamins may be lacking. For long-term use, supplemental vitamin capsules would be a good idea.

On the negative side (isn't there always one?) is the fact

that they are extremely boring and most people will not continue on the canned diets on a long-term basis. They are also unsatisfying in that there is nothing to chew, which from a cultural and psychological point of view (and perhaps even a medical one) is an important consideration. Some users have also found that they produce watery stools, diarrhea, gas, and occasionally constipation. Finally, the canned diets are rather expensive.

In summary, although the canned 900-calorie diets will help shed pounds, it is still better to cut the calories by going on a weight-reducing diet utilizing normal foodstuffs.

5. *"Sweets before eats."* The manufacturers of Ayds, and other brands of a similar nature, try to convince us that by having some sugar (in the form of their candies) before we sit down to eat our meals, we will have less appetite and more willpower. It is true that one of the factors in feeling satiated is the blood sugar level. Ayds contain about 25 calories per candy. Two Ayds (50 calories) are not going to affect the blood sugar level sufficiently for your body to notice. Although there may be some psychological effects of having candy before a meal, there are certainly no physiological ones.

Before-meal candies are not recommended for dieting.

6. *Bulk-increasing preparations.* Another *one* (and a relatively minor one, at that) of the factors which tell us we have had enough to eat is the volume of food in our stomachs. Bulk preparations (Metamucil, Konsyl, etc.) swell up when they absorb water, and this is supposed to fool our stomachs into believing that it is now filled with food, and that we have had enough to eat. For a variety of reasons, this type of trickery does not work; our bodies are much too sophisticated to fall for this device. In addition, if sufficient bulk medication is taken, it will act as a laxative.

Bulk producers are not recommended for dieting.

7. *Preparations containing benzocaine.* Benzocaine is a local anesthetic. The theory is that if our taste buds are numbed, we won't be hungry. Unfortunately, appetite (at least for food) is not centered in our mouths, but rather in our brains. Usually, these preparations (Slim-Mint, etc.) are combined with a bit of sugar and a bulk producer—indicating that the manufacturer does not have much confidence in the benzocaine, either.

Some of the benzocaine preparations are designed to numb you in the stomach if they don't succeed in the mouth. Dexule, Pondosan, Reducets, Wey-Dex, etc. are either in tablet or capsule form and are supposed to numb your stomach into believing you are not hungry. How silly.

None of the benzocaine products is recommended for dieting.

8. *OTC preparations containing amphetamine-like drugs.* This is the class of medicine most like the diet pills a doctor would be likely to prescribe. However, because they can be bought without prescription, the dose is much lower than a doctor would use. This reduces the effectiveness of the medication to the point that it probably will have only a psychological effect on appetite.

Three popular products in this category are Diet-Trim (which also contains benzocaine, the local anesthetic), Hungrex (which is wholly composed of the amphetamine-like drug), and Slender-X (which also has a bulk producer).

As indicated, if taken in the dose recommended, they are probably ineffective. However: if taken to excess, all the problems connected with the diet pills prescribed by doctors will apply here as well, except that there will not be a physician to supervise their use.

No OTC amphetamine-like preparations are recommended for dieting purposes, unless taken under the supervision of a physician.

9. *Diuretics (water pills).* Diuretics are valuable medicines for certain medical conditions such as heart failure, kidney disease, etc., and they are frequently prescribed by physicians. However, pills which cause a loss of water and therefore of body weight have no place in the self-treatment of overweight problems. Any temporary reduction in weight by this means will be quickly regained when the medicine is discontinued. To use diuretics on a chronic basis can be quite dangerous and should definitely be avoided, unless you are supervised by a physician. For self-treatment purposes, their only use should be for premenstrual tension, as mentioned in Chapter 15.

No OTC diuretics are recommended for dieting purposes, unless recommended by a physician.

Recommendations for Losing a Pound Per Week

1. Develop a regular exercise program. It does not have to be much; brisk walks for a half-hour twice a day, bicycling, swimming, or calisthenics are all satisfactory. It should be done on a regular basis and not performed to the point of fatigue or overexertion. If any medical problem exists, such as heart disease, high blood pressure, arthritis, etc., check with your doctor before beginning the exercise program. At any rate, start off slowly and build up the exercise program gradually.
2. If you are an average person with usual activities during your normal work and leisure time, aim for a diet consisting of about 1,200 calories per day. Ask your doctor for a weight-reducing diet or buy one at the drugstore. Ask the druggist for one recommended by doctors and *stay away from fad diets.*

   This is where most people get discouraged. However, it is not necessary to be precise in your calorie counting. You can approximate the intake of about 1,200 calories per day by doing the following:

   A. Eat balanced meals three times a day.
   B. Avoid all foods and meat with a high fat content, such as hamburgers, highly "marbled" steaks and other meats, sausages, etc. Preferred meats are chicken, fish, and veal.
   C. Avoid all fried and greasy foods (French-fried potatoes, onion rings, etc.).
   D. Stay away from the "trimmings" such as butter and sour cream on baked potatoes, sauces and gravies made with butter, oils, and fats.
   E. Do not eat processed or "junk" foods. Processed foods usually have a high concentration of calories and are low in other nutritive elements.
   F. Avoid sweets, cakes, pastries, milk shakes, nuts, ice cream, etc. except for special occasions.
   G. Stay away from nondiet drinks (Pepsi-Cola has 150 calories per 12-oz. glass).
   H. Alcohol is very high in calories and it is almost impossible to lose weight when drinking. Even beer has 110 calories per 8-oz. glass. The mixes used in highballs

(ginger ale, etc.) add significantly to the total calories. Soda water is the one exception in that it contains almost no calories.

I. *Do not snack*! Snacks are the easiest way to put on weight. Avoid bedtime and middle-of-the-night snacks. If you are hungry between meals have some tea or black coffee with a sugar substitute (if needed) and a couple of plain crackers.

J. Coffee and tea, without cream or sugar (or with a sugar substitute), contain no calories.

K. Do not engage in food fads or special diets, and do not employ special mechanical devices.

L. Supplemental vitamins and minerals are *not* necessary.

M. Overweight is a chronic problem. Dieting must be forever. Do not be discouraged. The weight will come off slowly, usually about a pound a week on the above schedule. When you have reached your preferred weight, you must continue to take precautions with your diet or you will put the weight right back on.

N. If you wish to count calories—and it is instructive to do so for a while—inexpensive booklets containing caloric values of commonly eaten foods are available at most drugstores.

O. Be aware of the fact that menstruating women will normally gain a few pounds a week or so before their period (due to retention of water), but this extra weight will be shed immediately after menstruation is over. Do not try to treat this weight gain.

P. Weight yourself only once a week, preferably at the same time (in the morning after urination is a good time), and on the same scale. Keep a written record.

OTC Medication for Weight Reduction

GROUP I
Not Recommended

A. Examples of amphetamine-like OTC preparations for weight reduction which are ineffective and/or potentially dangerous
   Adrinex
   Anorexin
   Appedrine

Dexatrim
Diet-Trim
Grapefruit Diet Plan Tablets
Hungrex
Pernathene-12
Prolamine
Slender-X
X-11 Reducing Plan

B. Examples of OTC diuretics (water pills)
Aqua-Ban
Diuretics (water pills)
Diurex Day-Span Water Capsules
Diurex Water Pills

C. Preparations containing benzocaine (local anesthetic)
Dexule
Diet-Trim
Figure Aid
Pondosan
Reducets
Slim-Line
Slim-Mint
Wey-Dex

Chapter 15

Menstrual Disorders

Menstruation has been the cause of concern for many women (and their doctors) since the beginning of recorded history. It is still a cause of concern for many. Some of the symptoms that may occur around the menstrual period are:

1. Pain
2. Weight gain and swelling
3. Premenstrual tension, headaches, and backaches
4. Bleeding between periods and irregular periods
5. Heavy bleeding during the period
6. Little or no bleeding

From the point of view of self-treatment and OTC drugs, only pain, weight gain and swelling, and premenstrual tension can be considered. If there is bleeding between periods, or excessive bleeding or scanty bleeding at the time of menstruation, or failure to bleed at the appropriate time, consult your doctor.

Menstrual Pain

Menstrual pain (also called dysmenorrhea) may be divided into two categories.

1. *Secondary dysmenorrhea.* This is a result of a definable abnormality in or around the female organs. In such instances, the pain is usually (but not always) dull, aching, steady, and frequently felt on one or both sides of the pelvis. It may extend to the low back and thighs, as well. This type of pain is characteristically due to infection or other medical problems such as endometriosis (tissue from the lining of the uterus located in abnormal positions). Because menstrual pain may be a symptom of an underlying

medical condition, all cases of painful menses should be checked by a doctor. This is especially true if severe menstrual pain begins after about age 20.

2. *Primary dysmenorrhea.* This accounts for the vast majority of women who complain of painful periods. The medical examination is normal, but pain is present. The characteristics of the pain are usually (but again, not always) somewhat different than in secondary dysmenorrhea. The pain in primary dysmenorrhea is usually sharp, cramping, intermittent, and most pronounced in the middle and lower abdomen. It is occasionally experienced in the low back, and less frequently in the vagina or thighs. The pain usually starts either before or during the period. Only very rarely does pain occur after the blood flow has ceased.

The cramps usually last from a few seconds to several minutes, with intervals of from a few minutes to half an hour or more between pains. Painful menstruation may be accompanied by nausea, vomiting, headache, backache, nervousness, irritability, joint pain, frequent and sometimes painful urination, or diarrhea. About half the women who experience severely painful menstrual cramps report that the pain lasts for less than one day; one-third of the women have severe pain for two days.

Menstrual pain occurs only in women who are ovulating—that is, releasing eggs each month in the middle of the cycle. The release of eggs is sometimes associated with another symptom known as "mittelschmerz." This German expression means "pain in the middle (of the cycle)." It refers to a mild form of pain that is sometimes felt on one side or the other of the lower abdomen. Timing is almost always just in between menstrual periods. It is due to release of the egg and is not normally associated with bleeding. In a few women, the pain can be pronounced, but most women either never experience "mittelschmerz" or notice only a slight discomfort at these times. Lack of this "in-between pain" does not mean a woman is *not* ovulating.

It is normal for women to have varying degrees of discomfort about the time of the period, but painful periods do not usually begin until several years after the onset of menstruation. This is so because ovulation, or the release of eggs, frequently does not occur for the first two or three years (or longer) after menstruation begins. Since painful menstruation is associated with periods in which ovulation occurs, it is usually not until the middle or late teens that pain may become a problem. The pain persists, if present, until the early or middle 20s and then begins to subside. However, giving birth almost always "cures" painful periods, presumably because the birth canal has been stretched.

How often women suffer from incapacitating painful periods is not precisely known, but menstrual cramps are one of the most common complaints in a gynecological practice. Probably somewhere between 10 and 20 percent of menstruating women who are childless suffer from severe and sometimes incapacitating menstrual pain.

Causes of Menstrual Pain

1. *Hormonal.* Hormones are chemicals made by glands and organs in the body that control many body functions. They signal when it is time to release the egg, to prepare the uterus (womb) for holding the fertilized egg, and, if fertilization has not occurred, to return the womb to its original state so the process can start again. The extra tissues which the uterus made to hold and nourish the egg must be sloughed off or discarded if fertilization does not occur. This sloughing-off of the womb's lining *is* menstruation. As an aid in expelling the unused and unneeded lining, contractions of the womb occur. It is analogous to birth except that instead of delivering a baby, the womb delivers the unused lining of its wall. The contractions are similar to those of childbirth, except, of course, they are much milder. Certain women, however, have severe pain as a result of menstrual contractions. This may be due to certain dynamics of the contraction process and to the anatomy of the womb, but this is not definitely proved. In any event, it is basically the contractions of the uterus, caused by hormonal influences, that are responsible for menstrual cramps.

2. *Psychological factors.* There is no doubt that psychological factors play a role in almost all cases of severe menstrual cramping. Every experienced physician is aware of this fact, and many scholarly works have been written on this subject. It appears that women with a conscious (or unconscious) fear of menstruation, or problems with other aspects of womanhood, are more likely to suffer severe

FIGURE 6
Female Reproductive System

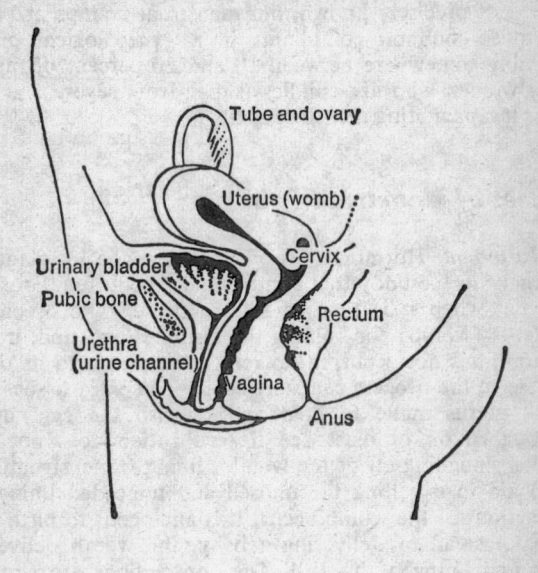

symptoms before or during the menstrual period. Often it is the manner in which a woman was raised and her attitudes toward sexuality and menstruation that are important in the development and the severity of symptoms. Menstrual difficulties, in fact, have a tendency to run in families. Even the language that is used to describe menstruation reflects distaste (what is there to like?). Terms such as "the curse," "*that* time of the month," "indisposed," "sick," "unwell," etc. are frequently used as cultural indicators of the repugnance that is associated with menstruation. Incidentally, neither menstruation nor the terms used to describe it are as tainted with displeasure in most other countries of the world.

To illustrate how important psychological factors are in relation to unbearable menstrual cramps, one study reported on the effect of weekly group-therapy sessions for six high school seniors who were disabled each month because of menstrual pain. They were all "cured" of their severe cramps after only three months! Although this "cure" may not have been permanent, it does indicate that pain and psychological factors can be tightly interwoven.

Very few gynecologists would suggest that unbearable menstrual pain is due only to psychological factors, but most would agree that the attitude and psychological makeup of the sufferer is an important component in the development of menstrual cramping.

3. *Miscellaneous factors.* There are a variety of miscellaneous factors which contribute to the production of severe menstrual cramps. A woman's pain threshold and pain response are very important. Cultural, socio-economic, and perhaps racial factors are also relevant.

Some women with intrauterine devices (IUD) report that menstrual cramps became more severe, but others with an IUD report that pain is less of a problem than before insertion.

Suggested Treatment Plan for Menstrual Cramps

1. Check with your doctor to be certain that they are not due to an underlying medical problem, particularly if the cramps begin after age 20.

2. For mild to moderate menstrual cramps:
   a. Plain aspirin, two or three tablets with a full glass of water or with meals, three or four times a day
   B. Heating pad applied to lower abdomen
   C. Moderate exercise sometimes helps (walking, bicycling, swimming).
3. If the simple measures above do not help, ask your doctor for codeine. This will almost always relieve difficult menstrual cramps so that they will not be incapacitating.
4. If all else fails, your doctor may wish to place you on birth-control pills or other hormones. Since this prevents ovulation (the release of an egg), and since ovulation is usually a prerequisite for menstrual cramps, the use of such medication very often alleviates the problem. It has been reported that when birth-control pills are used for three or four months and then stopped, incapacitating cramps frequently do not return.
5. For menstrual cramps that are intractable to the usual forms of therapy, psychotherapy has been of help in selected cases.

OTC Medication Available for Menstrual Cramps

No medication is recommended except plain aspirin. If aspirin cannot be tolerated, acetaminophen (Tylenol, etc.) may be used in the same dosage as aspirin.

Premenstrual Tension, Edema, and Weight Gain

It is "normal" for almost all menstruating women to have certain symptoms beginning seven to ten days before the menstrual period. These symptoms may include one or more of the following:

1. Edema (swelling), usually of hands, ankles, and face
2. A sense of "bloating"
3. Weight gain from 2 to 10 pounds
4. Irritability, emotional outbursts, crying spells, and depression
5. Fatigue

Menstrual Disorders

6. Difficulty in concentration
7. Headache (sometimes migraine headache)
8. Backache
9. Painful and swollen breasts
10. Increased appetite
11. Increased energy
12. Increased sexual appetite

These symptoms are extremely variable; some women have none, others have many. The symptoms may also change from month to month, although they are more likely to be relatively consistent. When premenstrual symptoms appear, they tend to be noticed approximately a week before the onset of the period, although some women experience them two weeks before and others only a day or two preceding the flow. Characteristically, they disappear within a day or two following the onset of the period. Unlike painful periods, they are not "cured" by childbirth and, in fact, have no correlation with menstrual cramps.

A woman, of course, is aware of all her symptoms; her husband, co-workers, and friends, more than likely, become aware only of the ones relating to her emotions. The emotional difficulties of women about the time of their menses is a very real phenomenon. In fact, the law in many countries recognizes that emotional instability is more prevalent before the menstrual period. In one study, it was determined that 62 percent of the crimes committed by inmates in a United States women's prison occurred during the week preceding the menstrual period. Other studies have indicated that suicide among women is more common in the premenstrual week than at any other time of the month.

Causes of Premenstrual Tension, Edema, and Weight Gain

The hormone changes that occur in a woman's body preceding the onset of menstruation are responsible for a number of physiological changes. One of the effects of the hormone activity at this time is the failure of the body to eliminate much of the salt that is ingested. In order to prevent an unhealthy concentration of salt, the body also retains water in the tissues to dilute the excess salt. This results in bloating, swelling, and weight gain. Some women have a sensation of bloating or fullness, others notice swelling in the ankles, face, hands, and breasts. When this occurs the scale usually verifies the suspicion of water retention by indicating a weight gain varying from 2 to 10 pounds.

Following the onset of the menstrual period, there is a return of hormone balance and loss of the excess water and salt that had been previously retained, with a return to normal weight.

The causes of the other symptoms of premenstrual tension are not as well understood. These symptoms may be related to edema of the brain and other body organs, but other theories attribute them to hormones, toxins, psychological factors, etc. There is no agreement of opinion concerning the reasons for premenstrual symptoms other than edema and weight gain.

Although the methods for self-treatment of premenstrual edema and tension are limited, they are often quite effective. The basic approach is to reduce salt intake and eliminate excess water in the premenstrual week. This is accomplished by restricting salt in the diet and/or using diuretics, which are drugs that help eliminate excess water. This will result in weight loss and reduce swelling, but will have variable effects on the other premenstrual symptoms. Salt restriction (and therefore lessened water accumulation) seems to decrease the emotionality and other mental symptoms in some women, but not in others. However, if premenstrual symptoms are troublesome, this form of treatment is worth trying. Although salt restriction is an effective means of reducing water accumulation, water restriction will not accomplish the same result unless done to extreme. So, drink normally, but reduce salt intake if premenstrual edema and tension are a problem.

It should be emphasized that one must not treat symptoms merely because they are present. If slight bloating, swelling, and weight gain are not very uncomfortable, or if they are not significantly affecting your life, there is no need to treat the symptoms at all. Likewise, if there is little, if any, difficulty with concentration, depression, etc., there is no need to attempt to relieve the last vestige of any symptom. It is far better to "live with" minor symptoms than to embark on an uncertain treatment program. It must be kept in mind that *all* medicines have potential side effects.

Suggested Treatment Plan for Premenstrual Tension, Edema, and Weight Gain

1. Limit table-salt intake beginning 10 to 14 days before the next menstrual period. Do not use medicines containing salt, such as sodium bicarbonate, Rolaids, Titralac, etc. (see Chapter 4). Try the salt-limitation program for two or three cycles. If it does not appreciably help, try the next steps.
2. Continue to limit salt, as above, but add a diuretic such as Pre-Mens Forte, one tablet, three or four times a day. Begin seven days before the onset of the period and discontinue one or two days after the onset of flow.
3. If the above program of salt restriction and diuretics is ineffective for three cycles, see your physician. He can prescribe additional and/or stronger medication that may help.

OTC Menstrual Products

OTC preparations for menstrual disorders do not distinguish between menstrual cramps and premenstrual tension. In various combinations they contain painkillers, diuretics, antihistamines, stimulants, and "uterine relaxers." The only ingredients that seem to have a rational place in the treatment of menstrual disorders are painkillers for cramps and diuretics for premenstrual bloating, swelling, and weight gain. Antihistamines are included in these products because of their sedative effect. This is the same class of drug used in OTC sleep-aids and anti-tension medicines. Caffeine is the most common stimulant used in these preparations, presumably to help get over the premenstrual blues. (Caffeine is also a mild diuretic.) A cup of coffee will be just as effective. Some products (Femicin) contain both a sedative and a stimulant! The "uterine relaxers" would seem to be a rational medicine for menstrual cramps. Unfortunately, none of the products available for OTC use is effective in relaxing the uterus. It would seem once again that the preparations available OTC for menstrual disorders are mostly irrational and ineffective, and, in susceptible persons, they may produce unwanted consequences.

The combination of medicines, which is foolishly intended

to affect all symptoms related to the menstrual cycle, is the most irrational feature of the OTC menstrual products. As has been pointed out, the treatment of menstrual cramps is primarily with the use of painkillers (as well as with heat, exercise, etc.), but there is no need for painkillers when the symptoms of premenstrual tension are foremost. Why use aspirin for emotional outbursts or other symptoms of premenstrual tension? Yet the most popular OTC menstrual product, Midol, contains aspirin as well as caffeine (equivalent to a single cup of coffee), plus a "uterine relaxer" (which has never been shown to be effective at all).

As for premenstrual tension, the only medicine available OTC which has any reasonable basis is a diuretic. These are listed in the accompanying tables.

OTC Products for Premenstrual Tension

GROUP I
Recommended Diuretics

These products also contain caffeine.

Name	Approximate Cost
Aqua-Ban	80 tablets for $2.98*
Pre-Mens Forte	48 tablets for 3.75

GROUP II
Not Recommended

Examples of preparations containing unnecessary, ineffective, and/or potentially harmful ingredients

Name	Comment
Femcaps Capsules	Aspirin, phenacetin, stimulants
Femicin	Antihistamine
Midol	Aspirin
Pamprin	Phenacetin, antihistamine
Sunril	Antihistamine
Trendar	Antihistamine

* Best buy in group.

Chapter 16

Insomnia and Tension

Insomnia

Attempting to convince your doctor that you must have a "good eight hours' sleep" is going to be difficult, since he, your doctor, probably functions quite well on considerably less.

The amount of sleep an individual requires varies greatly with age, activity, habit, and other factors. There is no "recommended" number of hours of sleep required. Some adults do very well on five or six hours, and others "need" eight or nine. The quality of sleep is also important. Some mornings we awaken with a feeling that we had a good night's rest and thus feel refreshed, but at other times, with the same hours of sleep, we may feel tired and groggy. Thus, no formula for the amount of sleep will be applicable to all persons, or even to the same person at different times. Unless lack of sleep occurs over a prolonged period of time, it is not harmful to your health.

Insomnia, or chronic difficulty in sleeping, may be indicated by trouble in falling asleep, frequent awakenings, early-morning awakening with inability to return to sleep, or a combination of these. We all have occasional difficulty in falling asleep, but only when getting to sleep and staying asleep is a problem over several weeks is the term "insomnia" applied.

Sleep is perhaps our most personal possession. When it is disturbed it is usually because something within our own heads is interfering with its normal rhythm. Internal causes of sleep loss include:

1. Emotional worries and stress, such as business and financial concerns, or other day-to-day worries of all sorts
2. Anticipation of events such as a trip or an examination
3. Depression, sadness, or agitation, whether concerned with immediate events (such as a recent death in the family) or one of long-standing and possibly vague origin

Even when we are at peace with ourselves, the world outside may seem to conspire to keep us awake. Such external causes of sleep loss include:

1. Excessive amounts of caffeine (a stimulant), as a result of ingestion of tea, coffee, cocoa, and cola drinks (Pepsi-Cola, Coca-Cola, etc.)
2. Drugs, especially those for control of obesity and weight problems (Preludin, Tenuate, etc.), because their stimulant action will make falling asleep difficult
3. Environmental problems such as a strange or uncomfortable bed, a room which is either too hot or too cold, or insects
4. Naps during the day

Medical Causes of Sleep Loss

Occasional difficulty with falling asleep, or staying asleep, is of little concern, and is usually due to one or more of the causes listed above. However, when the problem is chronic and there is trouble with the sleep pattern for several weeks (or more) at a time, there may be a more serious medical or psychological problem present, and this is when your physician should be consulted. Chronic insomnia may be caused by:

1. *Physical abnormalities*
   A. Pain
   B. Nighttime cough
   C. Frequent urination
   D. "Night cramps" in legs and feet
   E. Difficulty in breathing
   F. "Heartburn" or indigestion
   G. Itching (this may also be psychological)

2. *Psychological states.* Chronic depression or anxiety is extremely common and probably accounts for most cases of chronic insomnia. Paradoxically, treatment of this common cause of insomnia is not with "sleep-aids" or other sedatives but frequently with "psychic energizers." This class of medication helps to overcome depression and thus allows sleep to occur, but is available only by prescription.

Treatment of Insomnia with OTC Drugs

If there is occasional difficulty in either falling or remaining asleep, it is best to search for a cause of the disturbance and correct it if possible, before resorting to drugs. For instance, it is amazing how many cases of "insomnia" can be cured by the elimination of caffeine before retiring. Sipping cola in the evening, which contains a high concentration of caffeine, is a frequent cause of difficulty in falling asleep. Although TV may be a strong stimulus to dozing, the caffeine may be sufficient to keep you awake.

Understanding that sleep patterns change even in the same individual from time to time may help reduce anxiety over occasional changes in sleep rhythms. As people age, for instance, their need for sleep frequently diminishes. There are exceptions to this, but generally the elderly require fewer hours of sleep each day than the middle-aged or the young. Furthermore, the elderly, with less to do, often take little naps during the day, making their sleep requirements at night even less. They may therefore have difficulty falling asleep or staying asleep. Eliminating daytime naps may be all that is required to cure this form of "insomnia."

If a careful look at your habits and daytime activities fails to indicate the cause of your occasional sleep problem, or if your sleep difficulty is due to a known cause such as worry or anxiety that is not easily overcome, occasional OTC sleep-aids may be helpful.

On the other hand, whether or not you understand the cause of the sleep difficulty, if it is severe enough to interfere with your usual *daytime* activities, you should consult your doctor. If any of the situations listed under "Medical Causes" above apply to you, there is also need to see your doctor, since the insomnia may be a symptom of a more serious underlying medical or psychological condition.

OTC Sleep-aids

The vast majority of OTC sleep-aids contain one or more of the following drugs:
1. Bromides
2. Scopolamine

3. Miscellaneous drugs, such as aspirin and other pain-killers
4. Antihistamines

They are all associated with side effects, and except for antihistamines, none has any place in OTC sleep-aids. In fact, in 1975, the Federal Food and Drug Administration's panel on sleep-aids recommended that bromides, scopolamine, and the miscellaneous drugs be removed from the sleep-aid market. This is yet to be accomplished and you may continue to buy these potentially harmful drugs over the counter if you are not careful.

1. *Bromides.* Bromides have significant side effects that may include severe mental disturbances if taken for a prolonged period of time. On the other hand, a single dose of bromide is not effective in producing sleep because it takes several days for the concentration of this drug to build up sufficiently to cause drowsiness. Bromides have been more popular in years past, but are still contained in some OTC sleep preparations (Alva-Tranquil) and should definitely be avoided.

2. *Scopolamine.* Scopolamine is a drug used primarily to dry up secretions and it is frequently used for this purpose prior to surgery. However, there is *no* evidence that in the doses used in OTC sleep preparations it has any action as a sleep-aid. In spite of this, it is used in several popular products (Nite Rest, San-Man, Sominex, etc.).

   It is bad enough that scopolamine does not help the user get to sleep, but worse, it also has very significant side effects. Mental disturbances, dryness of mouth, blurred vision, and heart effects are the most common adverse reactions. It can be very dangerous if used by persons having certain forms of glaucoma (of which there are many unaware victims), prostate trouble, and heart disease. Scopolamine should be completely avoided in OTC drugs of *any* kind.

3. *Miscellaneous drugs.* Salicylamide, a weak aspirin-like drug, is a frequent ingredient of OTC sleep-aid medication (Nytol, Sominex, etc.), and it is difficult to justify its inclusion. Of course this has not prevented it from being marketed widely in these preparations. Should one ask a drug manufacturer why this class of medication is included

in sleep-aids, he would probably suggest that some cases of insomnia are due to pain. Although it is true that pain is an infrequent cause of insomnia, it would seem more rational to treat the pain with a more effective painkiller (such as plain aspirin), in which case no sedative at all would be needed. Salicylamide is a weak pain reliever, but it does possess significant side effects in susceptible persons. Even if it were harmless, which it is not, and even if it were an effective painkiller, which it is not, it does not make sense to put it in sleep-aids for general consumption when only a very small percentage of insomniacs would benefit from it. As has become apparent in other chapters in this book, this kind of irrational compounding of drugs is rampant in the OTC drug market. Watch out for it and do not be caught up by this kind of ill-conceived medication.

Other drugs and chemicals are also used in OTC sleep-aids, none of which has any rational use or proved effect as a sleep-inducer. These include vitamins, "passion flower" extract, and others.

4. *Antihistamines.* In general, the more effective the medicine, the less likely it is to be approved for OTC use. This is certainly true for sleep-aid medicines. For true insomnia, potent medication is available, but only by prescription from your doctor. The OTC drug manufacturers are careful to indicate that their products are for "occasional difficulty" in falling asleep or remaining asleep. They do not claim their products are the answer to insomnia, but this restraint is not entirely self-imposed; the Food and Drug Administration has "convinced" them to be circumspect in their advertising. The public, however, does not take in these advertisements literally, and the general assumption is that the products widely advertised on TV for sleep problems are effective for the relief of insomnia. Since the most effective drugs for serious sleep problems are by prescription only, there is but a single category of drugs available to the OTC market which has any degree of effectiveness as a sleep-aid: antihistamines.

It is of interest that antihistamines have no specific action on sleep. Their effectiveness is solely due to the side effect of drowsiness. That's right—the side effect of the medication (which ordinarily would be lessened or eliminated when used for other purposes) is employed here as the therapeutic tool. As one can imagine, the antihistamines with the greatest drowsiness side effects must be used if marketed for the purpose of sleep induction.

Because of the interaction of antihistamines with other drugs and their potential side effects other than drowsiness, the Food and Drug Administration's panel on OTC drugs, in 1975, suggested that all sleep-aid medications carry the following warnings:

A. "Do not take this product if you are presently taking a prescription or OTC drug without consulting a physician or pharmacist."
B. "If condition persists for more than 2 weeks consult your physician. Insomnia may be a symptom of serious underlying illness."
C. "For adults only. Do not give to children under 12 years of age."
D. "Take this product with caution if alcohol is being consumed."
E. "*Caution*: This product contains an antihistamine drug."

This is all good advice. You should not take a sleep-aid without a physician's advice if you are taking any other drug because the antihistamine may react with other drugs such as tranquilizers, hypnotics, etc.

If the sleep disorder lasts for more than two weeks it might be a reflection of another underlying problem and your doctor should be notified.

Children may be particularly susceptible to the sleep effect of antihistamines and thus antihistamines should not be used without a doctor's advice.

The depressant effect of alcohol and that of antihistamines are additive and the combination may result in "deeper sleep" than you bargained for.

You should be aware that the sleep-aid you may be using contains antihistamines because, however irrational, they are also used in other OTC preparations such as in cold medications. You may therefore be taking considerably more antihistamines with their attendant side effect of drowsiness than you intended. If you take sleep-aids in conjunction with either prescription antihistamines or OTC preparations containing antihistamines such as some cold tablets (see Chapter 1), you may get very sleepy indeed; not a happy situation if you are driving a car or working around machinery.

Insomnia and Tension

Additional Notes Concerning Antihistamines

1. Some persons are particularly susceptible to the drowsiness effect, even in recommended dosage.
2. Antihistamines have been used in suicide attempts by unstable persons.
3. Their effect is less predictable in the aged; the side effects are more likely to be serious.
4. Only about one-quarter of the sleep sufferers who try OTC sleep-aids will have any benefit from them.
5. When they do work, the drowsiness produced by sleep-aids does not wear off the moment you awaken in the morning but may persist well into the day. This may result in a considerable "hangover" in susceptible persons. It may also be particularly dangerous in people who take other drugs during the day, such as cold preparations containing antihistamines or alcohol.
6. A tolerance to the drug develops in a short while, so that even if it is effective at first, its benefits soon decrease. When this occurs, a "rebound" phenomenon may result in which it becomes more difficult than ever to fall asleep or to stay asleep.
7. Recently (1976) the FDA allowed the doubling of the dose in certain OTC antihistamines sold as sleep-aids. This will certainly improve the effectiveness of the drug but it is just as certain that it will significantly increase the side effects and possible dangers of these sleep-aids.

Side Effects of Antihistamines

1. They may be habit-forming.
2. Drying of mucous membranes in mouth and throat frequently occurs.
3. They may promote an inability to concentrate.
4. They may also promote:
    A. Dizziness and incoordination
    B. Ringing in the ears
    C. Blurred vision
    D. Nervousness
    E. Tremors

F. Loss of appetite, nausea, and vomiting
G. Heart palpitation

Of course, not all these side effects will occur in all cases or even in most cases. Some, or a combination of them, will occur in particularly susceptible users or if used to excess.

Cautions in the Use of Any Sleep-Aid

1. Do not exceed the recommended dosage.
2. Do not use on a regular basis. Sleep-aids should be limited to "occasional" use, i.e., no more than two or three times a week.
3. When using sleep-aids, do not take cold medicines, pain relievers, or any other drugs containing antihistamines. Be particularly careful about alcohol consumption.
4. Advise your doctor you are using sleep-aids if he prescribes any drug, but particularly sedatives, tranquilizers, or other sleep medications.

Suggested Treatment Plan for Mild Sleep Disorders

1. Avoid caffeine-containing liquids after 7:00 p.m. (coffee, tea, cocoa, cola drinks).
2. Do not nap during the day.
3. Do not use alcohol as a "nightcap."
4. Do not "force" sleep. If you have trouble falling asleep, do not fight it. Get up and read or watch TV until sleepy. Do not be worried about getting enough sleep. You will sleep when your body requires it.
5. If you get up and can't get back to sleep, read or watch TV. *Do not* just lie there and worry about not sleeping.
6. For occasional difficulty in falling asleep, you can use OTC sleep-aids listed in Group I. Use one or two capsules before retiring. Do not use more than two or three times a week.
7. If sleep difficulty becomes chronic—i.e., becomes an inability either to fall asleep or to stay asleep that persists for

Insomnia and Tension

several weeks at a time—see your doctor. It may be due to a medical or psychological problem that requires treatment.

OTC Sleep-Aids

GROUP I
Recommended

These contain antihistamine only.

Name	Approximate Cost
Compoz	30 tablets for $3.00
Dormin	12 capsules for 1.25
Relax-U-Caps	50 capsules for 0.92*
Sedacaps	30 capsules for 1.26
Sleepinal	20 capsules for 1.98
Somnicaps (American Pharmaceutical)	36 capsules for 1.12
Tranquim	20 capsules for 1.98

GROUP II
Not Recommended

Group II includes both OTC sleep-aids and daytime sedatives. Note that *no* OTC preparation is recommended for daytime use.

A. Examples of preparations containing scopolamine and/or pain medication

Calm-Aids
Devarex
Nite Rest
Nytol
Quiet World
San-Man
Seedate
Sleep-Eze

* Best buy in group.

Sleep-Aid
Slumberette
Sominex
Sominex 2
Sure Sleep
Tranquilium
Tranquinol

B. Examples of preparations containing bromides and thus considered potentially dangerous

Alva-Tranquil 8-Hour Timed Release
Alva-Tranquil Regular
Nervine Effervescent (Miles Nervine)

Tension

The magnitude of the "tension problem" is indicated by the fact that more tranquilizers are prescribed and sold than any other form of prescription medication. There are obviously a lot of people who feel they cannot cope with the tensions and anxieties of everyday life without help. For the medical practitioner, the easy way to treat the patient who complains of nervousness or tension is to prescribe a pill that will decrease anxiety. In many instances tranquilization can be very helpful and would be considered proper treatment even by the most critical anti-drug advocate within the medical profession. On the other hand, there is no doubt that tranquilizers and daytime sedatives are overprescribed. Tranquilizers and other prescription drugs used in the relief of tension are effective medicines. But these are powerful drugs; that is why they are "prescription only." OTC drugs sold for the same purpose are quite another matter.

Aside from the most important question of whether they *should* be used, the fact of the matter is that OTC daytime sedatives are *not* effective in alleviating anxiety and tension. Drugs sold as "daytime sedatives" are usually of the same formula as those in nighttime sleep-aids. They contain bromides, scopolamine, antihistamines, painkillers, vitamins, and other miscellaneous ingredients. The discussion above in relation to sleep-aids is relevant, therefore, to the daytime sedatives; only the name has been changed to "confuse the innocent."

The major ingredient in daytime sedatives is antihistamine. As previously indicated, a major side effect of antihistamines is drowsiness and sleep. It is this side effect of the drug that is utilized when it is sold as a sleep-aid. However, there is no evidence that antihistamines produce a calming or anti-tension action other than that afforded by their drowsy effect. Over-the-counter daytime sedatives are sold for relief of "simple nervousness due to common everyday overwork and fatigue," "for the relief of occasional simple nervous tension," etc. The fact is that if they work at all, it is because they make the user drowsy. Prescription tranquilizers, on the other hand, have the property of reducing tension and anxiety without producing drowsiness, although this ideal is not always realized.

The sale of daytime sedatives is particularly onerous because the drowsiness they produce can be quite dangerous. It is one thing when antihistamines are used to induce drowsiness in people wishing to get to sleep. It is quite another when they are used during the day on the pretext of providing a "calming" effect and drowsiness is produced at the very time you wish to be most alert. Reduced alertness, inability to concentrate, incoordination, and reduced reflex time may occur with the use of this medication during the daytime hours.

Some of the daytime sedatives include aspirin and other mild painkillers on the theory that pain, particularly headache, is a common cause of tension. This is probably true, but why not take plain aspirin if a headache is present? It does not make sense to pay the price of drowsiness for the relief of headaches when aspirin will probably relieve the headache without producing this annoying and potentially dangerous symptom. As usual, TV advertising is far more potent than common sense.

To repeat, *no* OTC sedatives are recommended for daytime use.

Subject Index

Acne:
  in adults, 78
  and birth control, 78
  cause of, 76, 78
  and cleanliness, 79
  cleansers, 79
  and cosmetics, 78, 80
  and dandruff, 83
  description of, 76, 78
  diet for, 78, 79
  drying agents, 81, 82
  factors affecting, 78, 79, 80
  home treatment for, 79, 80
  hormones and, 78, 80
  OTC effectiveness, 76
  OTC ingredients for, 80, 81, 82
  OTC not recommended, 82
  soaps for, 80
Adenoids, 17, 21
Aerosols, 25
Alcohol:
  in cough preparations, 30, 31, 33
  and indigestion, 35, 38, 39
  and sleep-aids, 166, 167, 168
  and vitamin deficiencies, 135
  and weight loss, 148, 149
Allergic Rhinitis (see Allergy)
Allergy (see also Hay Fever):
  and antihistamines, 1, 9, 30
  and aspirin, 116
  cause of, 4, 98
  cosmetic, 78
  and diarrhea, 52
  eczema and, 88
  to plants, 98
  and sore throat, 20
  symptoms, 4, 25, 30
Ameba, 51

Anemia:
  and aspirin, 114, 116
  from hemorrhoids, 68, 71
  from stomach bleeding, 114, 116
  from vitamin deficiency, 134
Anesthetic:
  in burn preparations, 90, 94
  for cold sores, 87
  in cough drops, 19, 27, 31
  in diet aids, 146, 147, 150
  in hemorrhoid preparations, 72, 73, 75
  in liniments, 137, 138
  for plant poisoning, 100, 101
  sensitivity to, 19, 27, 73, 87, 90
  in throat lozenges, 19, 27, 31
Antacids:
  acid rebound, 41
  in aspirin, 42, 47, 112, 113, 120, 123, 130
  in cold remedies, 9
  and constipation, 41, 46, 58
  and diarrhea, 52
  how they work, 39, 40
  how to take, 42, 43
  for indigestion, 37, 40–47
  ingredients of, 40, 41, 42, 44–47
  and kidney stones, 41, 43
  OTC acceptable, 46
  OTC not recommended, 47
  OTC recommended, 43, 44, 45
  salt in, 159
  side effects, 40, 41, 42, 46
  simethicone, 42, 45
  sodium content of, 41, 43, 44

173

treatment plan with, 42, 43
Antibiotics:
  for acne, 80
  and burns, 91, 92, 95
  and diarrhea, 52
  effectiveness of, 1, 18, 27, 72
  in OTC preparations, 18, 19, 27, 31
  for strep throat, 19, 20
  and sun, 93, 94
  and viruses, 1, 18
Antidiarrheals, 52, 53, 54, 55
Antihistamines:
  for allergies, 1, 9, 30
  for colds, 1, 9, 14, 15, 166
  for cough, 30, 33, 34
  effects of, 9, 159, 165, 166, 170, 171
  for flu, 1
  for hay fever, 1, 9
  for headache, 121, 123
  for menstrual disorders, 159, 160
  for plant poisoning, 100, 101
  in sedatives, 170, 171
  side effects of, 9, 30, 165, 166, 167, 168, 170, 171
  in sleep-aids, 163, 164, 165, 166, 168, 169
  and sun, 94
  tolerance to, 167
Antiseptics:
  action of, 72
  for eye problems, 105, 106
  for hemorrhoids, 72, 74, 75
Anus (see also Hemorrhoids):
  and hemorrhoids, 67, 68
  itching, 69, 70, 74
  medicine application to, 73
  serious symptoms of, 69, 70
  sphinctor, 68
Appetite:
  and blood sugar level, 146
  exercise effect on, 142, 143, 148
  loss of, 2, 3, 128, 168
  premenstrual increase in, 156
  reduction by "dieting aids," 144, 145, 146, 147

reduction by medication, 144, 145
Arthritis (see also Gout, Osteo-arthritis, and Rheumatoid Arthritis):
  and age, 125, 127, 128, 129, 133
  drug of choice, 127, 128, 129, 130, 132
  drugs for and sun exposure, 94
  external remedies, 131, 136–138
  heredity and, 126, 127, 132
  in men vs. women, 126, 127, 128, 129, 132, 133
  and occupation, 125, 128
  and rest, 127, 128, 129, 130, 133
  symptoms of, 124, 126, 127, 128, 129, 131, 132, 133
  treatment for, 127, 128, 129, 130, 131, 136–138
  types of, 125–127, 128–129, 131–132, 133
Ascorbic Acid (see Vitamins)
Aspirin:
  absorption time of, 113
  and antacids, 42, 47, 112, 113, 120, 123, 130
  for arthritis, 127, 128, 129, 130, 136
  for burns, 90, 91
  for children, 114, 116
  and cold contagion, 7, 11
  for colds, 7, 9, 11
  cost of, 119, 120
  for cough, 30, 34
  dosage of, 7, 12, 19, 20, 113, 114, 115, 116, 127, 128, 130
  drug interaction, 117, 130
  for dismenorrhea, 156, 160
  how it works, 19
  how to take, 7, 19, 20, 112, 113, 114, 127, 128, 130
  for itching, 99
  in sedatives, 171

Subject Index

side effects of, 42, 112, 113, 114, 115, 116, 117, 123, 128, 130, 135
 in sleep aids, 164, 165
 for sore throat, 19, 20, 21
 timed-release, 113, 121
 "topical," 19, 113, 121
Asthma:
 from aspirin, 116
 and hay fever, 4
Astringents, 72, 74, 75, 81, 82, 86, 87
Atherosclerosis, 139

Backache:
 with flu, 2
 premenstrual, 151, 152, 157
Bacteria:
 culturing of, 19
 infections from, 1, 3, 6, 19, 25, 26
 pneumonia, 6, 25
 streptococcus, 1, 3, 19, 20
Blackheads:
 cause of, 76, 78
 description of, 76, 78
 treatment of, 79
Blisters:
 in burns, 89, 91
 cold sores, 86, 87, 93
 treatment of, 91
Blood:
 with hemorrhoids, 68, 69, 70, 71, 73, 74
 in sputum, 25
 in stool, 37, 52, 59, 68, 69, 70
 in vomitus, 37
Blood Pressure:
 and cold remedies, 12, 15
 decongestants, effects on, 8, 30
 drugs and sun exposure, 94
 and exercise, 148
 and headache, 117
 and overweight, 139
 and sodium, 41
Bowel (see also Stool):
 change in habits of, 57, 59, 62, 70

 diagram of, 36
 diseases of, 37, 57, 58, 59
 irritable colon, 57
 movements, 40, 46, 48–125
 mucous colitis, 50
 parts of, 36, 38, 48
 regularity of, 56, 57, 58
 transit time in, 48
 water reabsorption, 48, 56
Bronchitis, 25
Bulk-forming laxatives:
 action of, 60, 61
 dose of, 61, 63
 natural, 61, 63
 sample OTC products, 64
 and swallowing difficulty, 61, 63
 synthetic, 61, 63
Burns (see also Sunburn):
 aspirin for, 90, 91
 first degree, 89, 90, 91
 OTC not recommended, 90, 91, 95
 OTC recommended, 94, 95
 second degree, 89, 91
 third degree, 89, 90, 91, 92
 treatment of, 90, 91, 92
 types of, 89, 90

Caffeine:
 in antacids, 42
 in cold remedies, 9
 drinks containing, 43, 44, 162, 168
 and insomnia, 162, 168
 in menstrual disorder remedies, 159
 and stomach acid, 42, 43
Calories:
 and exercise, 142, 143
 fat conversion of, 141
 number needed, 141, 142, 145, 148
Cancer:
 early signals, 23, 26
 large bowel, 57, 58
 lung, 23, 26
 stomach, 35, 39
 and thyroid medication, 145

Subject Index

Canker Sores (see Cold Sores)

Cathartics:
- abuse of, 57, 58, 59, 63, 74
- action of, 61, 62
- contact, 61, 62, 65
- and diarrhea, 52
- salts as, 61, 62, 63, 65, 66
- side effects, 61, 62
- warnings in use, 61, 62
- when to use, 59, 63

Children:
- headache treatment, 114, 115, 120, 122
- medication warnings, 53, 54, 63, 64, 137, 166
- overweight in, 141

Cholera, 48

Cirrhosis, 68

Cold, common (see also Cold Remedies):
- causes of, 1, 5, 7, 9, 18
- cures for, 5, 11
- drugs for, 1, 5, 7, 8, 13, 24
- duration, 2, 6, 11, 12
- economic effects of, 5, 6
- fever in, 2, 12
- OTC not recommended, 9, 11, 12, 14, 15, 16
- other names for, 1
- preventatives for, 5, 9, 10, 11
- symptoms of, 1, 2, 7, 18, 20, 25, 26
- treatment of, 6, 7, 8, 11, 12
- vitamin C and, 9, 10, 11
- and weather, 5

Cold Remedies:
- antihistamines, 9
- aspirin, 7, 9, 12
- for children, 12
- decongestants, 7, 8, 9, 12
- ingredients of, 7-9
- phenacetin in, 9
- steam inhalation, 12
- vitamin C, 5, 9, 10, 11
- warnings in use, 9, 11, 12, 15

Cold Sores:
- cause of, 86
- contagion of, 86
- OTC medications for, 87
- reoccurrence of, 86
- sun effect on, 93
- treatment for 86, 87

Colon (see Bowel)

Compresses, cold:
- for burns, 90, 91
- for eye irritation, 106

Conjunctiva:
- description of, 102, 103
- reaction to irritation, 102
- trachoma, 104

Conjunctivitis, 102, 104

Constipation:
- and abdominal pain, 60, 63
- causes for, 41, 46, 50, 57, 58, 59
- defined, 57
- diseases causing, 58, 59
- drugs causing, 58, 59
- emotional distress and, 57
- foods to relieve, 58, 59, 60, 61, 63
- and hemorrhoids, 67
- irritable colon, 57
- OTC not recommended, 66
- OTC products lists, 64, 65, 66
- treatment guide, 62, 63
- types of OTC for, 60, 61, 62
- when to see the doctor, 59, 60

Contact Dermatoses (see Allergy and Poison Ivy)

Cortisone, 116

Cough:
- with blood or sputum, 12, 25, 26, 27, 28
- causes for, 25, 31
- in the common cold, 1, 2, 25, 26
- expectorants, 28, 29, 31, 32
- extra OTC ingredients, 29, 30
- with fever, 26
- with flu, 1, 2, 25, 26
- home remedies, 26, 27, 28, 31
- humidification, 27, 28
- nighttime, 162, 163

Subject Index

nonproductive, 26, 27, 28, 31
OTC for diabetics, 28, 29, 32
OTC not recommended, 32, 33, 34
OTC recommended, 31, 32
pills and tablets for, 29
productive, 26, 27, 30, 31
purpose of, 23
and serious disease, 23, 25, 26
and smoking, 23, 25, 26
suppressants, 27, 28, 29, 31, 32
in tonsillitis, 3
treatment of, 26, 27, 28, 31, 32
when to see the doctor, 25, 26, 31

Cough Drops:
for cough, 26, 27, 31
ingredients, 18, 19, 27, 31
OTC acceptable, 21
OTC not acceptable, 22
side effects, 18, 27

Cradle Cap, 83

Dandruff:
and acne, 83
and balding, 83
description of, 83
effective ingredients, 83, 85
OTC not recommended, 84, 85, 86
OTC recommended, 83, 84, 85
treatment plan, 83, 84

Decongestants:
in cold treatment, 7, 8, 9, 11, 13, 14
and cough, 30, 32, 33
dangers of, 8
effective dose of, 7, 13
for headache, 121, 123
how they work, 7, 8, 30
local vs. oral, 8, 13–14, 15, 16
OTC acceptable, 13, 14
OTC recommended, 13

OTC unacceptable, 14
phenylephrine, 7, 8
rebound effect of, 8, 13
side effects of, 8, 30

Depression:
and constipation, 59
and diet drugs, 145
drugs for and sun exposure, 94
and insomnia, 162
premenstrual, 156
treatment of, 162

Diabetes:
and arthritis, 132
aspirin and tests for, 116
and cold remedies, 12, 15, 16
and cough remedies, 29, 32
decongestants effects, 8
and diarrhea, 52
drug reaction with excessive sun, 94
and neuralgia, 134
and overweight, 139
vitamin C effects, 10

Diaphragm, 24

Diarrhea:
and abdominal pain, 50, 51, 52
bulk-formers, 53, 54, 55
causes, 48, 50, 51, 52
with colds, 2
diet for, 53
drug causing, 52
emotional causes, 50
food poisoning, 51
gelling agents, 52, 53, 54, 55
and hemorrhoids, 67
with menstruation, 152
OTC not recommended, 55
OTC recommended, 54, 55
and roughage, 53
in stomach flu, 50, 51
traveler's, 51
treatment of, 37, 52–54
from vitamin C, 10
and water content, 48, 50, 53
when to see the doctor, 52

Diet:
and acne, 78, 79

Subject Index

for arthritis, 124, 130
for constipation, 58, 59, 61, 63
for diarrhea, 53
for hemorrhoids, 70, 74
low sodium, 61, 63
OTC for overweight, 143, 144, 145, 146, 147, 148
pills, 144, 145, 147, 149, 150
premenstrual, 158, 159
Digestion, 38
Digestive System:
  abdominal pain, 50, 51
  bleeding in the, 68, 69
  diagram of, 36
  diseases of, 38
  food processing by, 48, 56
  organs of, 35, 36, 38, 48, 56
  pain in, 37, 38, 39
  tumors of, 68
Diuretics:
  for edema, 158, 159
  for overweight, 147, 150
  for premenstrual tension, 147, 158, 159, 160
  and sun reaction, 94
Diverticulitis, 37
Diverticulosis, 37
Dizziness:
  from antihistamines, 167
  from aspirin, 116, 128, 130, 135
Drowsiness:
  as a drug side effect, 9, 28, 30, 165, 166, 167
Dysentery:
  amebic, 51
  bacterial, 51
Dysmenorrhea:
  and age, 152, 153, 154
  characteristics of, 151, 152
  endometrics and, 151
  hormones and, 153, 156
  and intrauterine devices, 154
  and ovulation, 152, 156
  psychological factors, 153, 154, 156
  and serious disease, 151, 152
  treatment plan, 154, 156

Ear:
  ringing in, 114, 116, 128, 130, 135, 167
Earache:
  in strep throat, 3, 19, 20
  in tonsillitis, 3
Eczema:
  an allergic reaction, 88
  description of, 88
  and doctor's care, 88
  infantile, 88
  types of, 88
Edema (swelling):
  cause of, 158
  and diuretics, 158
  premenstrual, 156, 157, 158
Emphysema, 25
Endocrine system (see also Hormones)
  and constipation, 58
  and diarrhea, 52
Endometriosis, 151
Enema:
  misuse of, 58, 62, 63, 64, 66
  oil-retention, 62, 66
  OTC products, 66
  salt, 62, 66
  side effects of, 62
  tap water, 62, 63
Esophagus:
  diagram of, 36
  diseases of, 35, 38
  stomach and acid effects on, 37, 38, 39
Exercise:
  and appetite, 142, 143
  calories used in, 142, 143
  effects of, 142, 143
  programs, 148
  warnings for, 148
Eye (see also Conjunctiva):
  artificial tears, 107, 108, 109
  cleansing agents, 105, 106, 107
  diagram of, 103
  irritants, 105, 107
  migraine symptoms, 118
  OTC preparations, 107, 108, 109

Subject Index

OTC product storage, 106
pain in, 102, 104
parts of, 102
self-treatment of problems, 102, 104, 105, 106, 107
serious symptoms, 104, 105, 107
strain, 110, 117
symptoms with allergies, 4, 105
symptoms with colds, 2, 105
symptoms with flu, 2, 105
vasoconstrictors, 106, 108
Eye Cleansers, 105, 106, 107

Fainting, 25
Fasting:
and headache, 110, 117
Fever:
with arthritis, 128, 131, 133, 136
aspirin treatment for, 7, 117
with colds, 2, 12
with cough, 25
with flu, 2, 19
with hay fever, 4
with sinusitis, 4
with stomach flu, 50
with strep throat, 3, 19, 20
with tonsillitis, 3
Fever Blisters (see Cold Sores)
Flu:
duration of, 2, 51
other names, 2
stomach, 50, 51
symptoms of, 2, 7, 18, 19, 50, 51, 117
treatment of, 12
viral cause, 1, 2, 50

Gall Bladder:
diseases of, 37, 139
stones, 37, 139
Gargles:
OTC, 18, 21, 22
salt, 12, 18, 20
Gastroenteritis, acute (see Stomach Flu)

Glaucoma:
and decongestants, 8
drug warnings, 8, 164
symptoms of, 105
Gout:
and age, 133
and aspirin, 116
symptoms of, 131, 132, 133
treatment of, 132
Grippe (see Flu)

Hair:
diagram of, 77
and dandruff, 83–86
lubrication of, 76
Hay Fever:
and antihistamines, 1, 9
fever in, 4
symptoms of, 1, 4
Head (see also Headache)
cold symptoms in, 1
serious disease, 110, 118, 119
Headache:
causes of, 110, 117, 118
with colds, 1, 2, 7, 12, 110, 117
combination drugs for, 112, 113, 116
drugs of choice for, 112, 113, 114, 117, 118, 119, 120
as a drug side effect, 9
with flu, 2, 110, 117
migraine, 110, 118
OTC, 112, 113, 114, 115, 116, 119, 120, 122, 123
OTC unacceptable, 121, 123
premenstrual, 151, 152, 157
as a serious symptom, 110, 118, 119
with sinusitis, 4, 110, 118
with strep throat, 3
tension, 110, 111, 112, 113, 114
with tonsillitis, 3
treatment of, 111, 112, 113, 114, 115, 116
types of, 110, 117, 118, 119
Head Cold (see Cold, common)

Heartburn:
　vs. heart disease, 37, 39
　and insomnia, 162
　from stomach refluxing, 38
Heart Disease:
　and cold remedies, 12, 15, 16
　and constipation, 58, 60
　and cough, 25
　drugs for & sun exposure, 94
　vs. heartburn, 37, 39
　and hemorrhoids, 68, 71
　OTC drugs warnings, 12, 15, 16, 41, 43, 61, 63
　and overweight, 139
　and rheumatoid arthritis, 128, 129
　from strep infections, 19
　symptoms of, 25
Heat Stroke, 93
Heberden's Nodes, 126, 127, 133
Hemorrhoids:
　abdominal pressure and, 67
　and anemia, 68, 71
　bleeding with, 68, 69, 70, 71, 73, 74
　causes of, 67, 68
　cortisone for, 74
　and defecation, 59, 60, 67, 68, 69, 70, 71, 74
　description of, 67
　diet for, 70, 74
　heredity and, 67
　medication forms, 73
　occupation and, 67
　OTC ingredients, 72, 73
　OTC recommended, 74
　pregnancy and, 67, 71
　protrusion of, 68, 69, 70, 71, 72, 73, 74
　self-treatment, 70, 71, 73
　and stool softeners, 59, 60, 70, 71, 74
　symptoms of, 68, 69, 70, 71
　surgery for, 69, 71
　treatment plan, 73, 74
　types of, 68, 69, 73
　when to see the doctor, 69, 70, 71, 72, 73, 74

Heredity, role of:
　in acne, 78
　in arthritis, 126, 127, 132
　in dysmenorrhea, 154
　in hemorrhoids, 67
　in neuralgia, 134
　in overweight, 142
Hernia, 35, 38, 39, 59
Herpes (see Cold Sores, Viruses)
Hormones:
　and acne, 78
　and acne treatment, 80
　and menstruation, 153, 156, 157, 158
　and treatment of overweight, 145
Humidification:
　for colds, 12
　for coughs, 27, 28, 31
　for rooms, 17, 21, 27
　in sore throat, 17, 21
Hypertension (see Blood Pressure)

Ice:
　for burns, 90, 91
Indigestion (see also Heartburn):
　and antacids for, 37, 38, 39–44
　causes of, 35, 37, 38, 50
　chronic, 43
　liquid preparations, 42, 43, 44, 45
　milk for, 43
　other names for, 38
　OTC products, 43, 44, 45, 46
　OTC not recommended, 47
　self-treatment, 35, 37, 38, 39, 42, 43, 44
　and serious disease, 35, 37, 38, 39, 43, 44
　when to see a doctor, 37, 43, 44
Infections:
　bacterial, 1, 3, 6, 19, 25, 26
　lung, 25, 26

Subject Index

upper respiratory, 1–12, 18, 19, 20
viral, 1, 2, 3, 9, 18, 19, 20
Infectious Mononucleosis, 20
Influenza (see Flu)
Insomnia:
  characteristics of, 161
  from drugs, 30, 162
  drug warnings, 163, 164, 165, 166, 167, 168, 169, 170
  from emotional causes, 161, 162
  medical causes, 162, 163, 164, 166, 168
  OTC treatment of, 163, 164, 165, 166, 168, 169
  from stimulants, 162
  treatment plan, 168
Itching:
  cold sore, 86
  with dandruff, 83
  with eczema, 88
  of eyes, 104, 105
  hemorrhoidal, 69, 70, 74
  and insomnia, 162
  with poison ivy and oak, 98, 99
  with psoriasis, 87, 88
  rectal, 69, 70, 74
  treatment of, 99

Jaundice, 52, 70
Joints:
  cartilage replacement, 126
  deformity, 126, 128, 129, 133, 136
  pain with menstruation, 152
  wear and tear, 126
Joint Disease (see Arthritis, Neuritis, Neuralgia, and Rheumatism)

Kidney Disease:
  and cathartics, 61, 63
  and gout, 132
  and overweight, 139
  and rheumatic arthritis, 128, 129
  and sodium, 41, 43, 61
  stones, 41, 43
  from strep infections, 19, 21
  vitamin C effects, 10
Kidneys:
  damage and headache remedies, 117
  and water excretion, 48

Laxatives (see also Bulk-Forming Laxatives, Cathartics, Enemas, Rectal Suppositories, Salts, and Stool Softeners):
  abuse of, 57, 58, 63
  dosage of, 60, 61
  effect of, 58, 60, 61
  OTC products, 64–66
  and pregnancy, 64
  side effects of, 60, 61
  types of, 40, 41, 60, 61, 62
  warnings for use of, 61, 63, 64
  when to use, 59, 63
Liniments:
  action of, 131, 136, 137
  for arthritis, 131, 136, 137
  for neuralgia, 135, 136, 137
  OTC, 138
  warnings for use of, 131, 137
Lozenges, throat:
  for cough, 26, 27, 31
  ingredients, 18, 19, 27, 31
  OTC acceptable, 21, 22
  side effects, 18, 19, 27
  for sore throat, 18, 19
Lubricants, 70, 72, 74, 75
Lungs:
  diagram of, 24
  emphysema, 25
  infections of, 6, 25
  tumors, 25
Lupus Erythematosis, 93
Lymph Glands:
  enlargement of, 3, 19
  in strep throat, 3, 19, 20
  in tonsillitis, 3

Malaise:
  in colds, 2, 7

in stomach flu, 50, 51
in strep throat, 3
in tonsillitis, 3
Menstruation (see also Dysmenorrhea):
  and acne, 78
  bleeding irregularities, 151
  cramping, 152, 153, 154, 156, 157
  and diuretics, 147, 158–160
  edema and, 156, 157, 158, 159, 160
  OTC products for, 159, 160
  ovulation and, 152, 153, 156
  pain and, 151, 152, 153–156, 157
  premenstrual symptoms, 151, 152, 156, 157, 158–160
  treatment, 159–160
Migraine, 110, 118, 157
"Mono" (see Infectious Mononucleosis)
Mouth Breathing, 17, 18, 21
Mucous Colitis, 50
Mucous Membranes:
  antihistamines and, 1, 9, 30, 167
  decongestants and, 8, 106
  and smoking, 18
  and sore throat, 17, 18, 20
Mucus:
  with hemorrhoids, 68
  in stool, 50, 52, 59
  in vomitus, 37
Muscle:
  aching, 2, 7, 19, 135
  with arthritis, 127
  contraction headaches, 110, 111
  cramping, 162
  pain treatment, 135, 136, 137, 138
  wasting, 128, 129, 136

Nerves (see also Neuralgia):
  symptoms of, 134
  types of, 134
Nervousness (see also Tension):
  and coughing, 23
  and diarrhea, 48, 50
  and indigestion, 37, 39, 43, 44
Neuralgia:
  causes of, 134, 135
  symptoms, 134, 135
  treatment of, 135, 136, 137, 138
Neuritis (see Neuralgia)
Nose:
  decongestants, 7, 8, 12, 13, 14
  drops, 8, 12, 13–14
  spray, 8, 12, 13–14
  sunshades for, 92
  URI symptoms, 1, 2, 7, 8, 12, 19

Obesity (see also Appetite, Diet, and Weight):
  and acne, 79
  and age, 142
  and arthritis, 128, 130, 139
  causes of, 141, 142, 143
  definition of, 139
  diseases associated with, 139
  drug warnings, 145, 147
  effects of, 139
  hormones, 145
  OTC preparations for, 144, 145, 146, 147, 149, 150
  treatment programs, 143, 144, 145, 148, 149
Ointments, 72, 73, 74, 75
Osteoarthritis:
  and age, 125, 127
  causes of, 125, 126
  finger nodes, 126, 127, 133
  generalized, 126, 127, 133
  localized, 125, 126, 127, 133
  and occupation, 125, 128
  symptoms of, 126, 127, 133
  treatment of, 127, 128
  and vitamin C, 11
Overeating:
  and indigestion, 35, 38, 39
Overweight (see Diet, Obesity)
Ovulation, 152, 153, 156

Subject Index

Pain Killers (see Acetaminophen, Aspirin)
Pancreas:
  diseases of, 37
Parkinson's Disease, 58, 83
Pharyngitis (see Tonsillitis)
Phenacetin:
  in cold remedies, 9
  side effects, 9
Pimples:
  causes of, 76, 77, 78
  treatment for, 79, 80
Pink Eye, 106, 107
Pneumonia:
  and the common cold, 6
  and cough, 25
Poisoning, accidental:
  from liniments, 137
Poison Ivy:
  and allergy reaction, 88, 98
  geographical distribution, 98
  OTC ingredients, 100, 101
  OTC not recommended, 101
  OTC recommended, 100
  severe, 99
  susceptibility to, 98
  symptoms, 98, 99
  treatment, 99, 100, 101
Poisons:
  chemical, 134
  in food, 35
  and indigestion, 35
  plant, 98, 99
Poison Sumac (see Poison Ivy)
Pollen:
  allergy to, 4
Pores, skin:
  clogging of, 76, 78
  and cosmetics, 78, 80
  peel creams for, 79
Porphyria, 93
Pregnancy:
  drug warnings, 11, 116
  and dysmenorrhea, 153, 157
  hemorrhoids during, 67, 71
  and sun sensitivity, 93
Psoriasis:
  and arthritis, 88, 132
  description of, 87, 88
  treatment of, 84, 87, 88
Puberty:
  and acne, 76, 78
Pus:
  in eyes, 104
  on tonsils, 3

Rashes:
  with arthritis, 128, 129, 133, 136
  from aspirin, 116, 123
  drug reactions, 93, 116
  in eczema, 88
  in poison ivy, 88, 98
  in psoriasis, 88
  with strep infection, 19, 20
  streaking, 98
Rectal Suppositories:
  glycerin, 62
  for hemorrhoids, 73, 74, 75
  ineffectiveness, 73
  misuse, 62, 63
  OTC products, 66
  side effects, 62
Rectum:
  bleeding from, 68, 69
  and hemorrhoids, 67, 68, 69
  pain in, 70
  warning symptoms, 70
Reproductive System, female:
  diagram of, 155
  monthly cycle, 153
Respiratory Infections (see Flu, Infections)
Respiratory System:
  bronchitis, 25
  diagram of, 24
  emphysema, 25
  infections in, 1–12, 19, 20, 23, 25, 26
  pneumonia, 6, 25
Rheumatism (see also Arthritis):
  definition of, 124
  OTC for, 136, 138
Rheumatoid Arthritis:
  and age, 128, 129, 133
  finger nodes, 126, 127
  symptoms of, 128, 129, 133

Subject Index

systematic nature of, 128, 129, 133
treatment, 128, 130, 131
Rhus Plants, poisonous, 98

Salmonella, 51
Salt:
 for acne, 79
 compresses for burns, 91
 for diarrhea, 53
 diet restriction of, 158, 159
 for gargling, 12, 18, 20, 21
 premenstrual retention of, 158, 159
Salts:
 enemas, 62, 66
 laxative, 61, 63, 65, 66
 warnings, 61, 63, 64
Sebaceous Glands:
 and acne, 76, 78
 diagram of, 77
 and hair follicles, 76, 77
 iodine effects, 79
 sebum production, 76
Seborrhea (see also Dandruff), 83–86
 and Parkinson's Disease, 83
Sebum:
 and acne, 76, 78, 79
 iodine effects, 79
Sedatives (see also Sleep-Aids), 58, 166, 168
 OTC effectiveness, 170, 171
 OTC ingredients, 170, 171
 warnings against, 171
Sinusitis:
 cause of, 4, 118
 symptoms, 4, 110, 118
 treatment of, 118
Sitz Baths, 70, 71, 74
Sjögren's Syndrome, 107
Skin Cleansers, 79, 80, 82
 for burns, 90, 91, 92
Skin Problems:
 acne, 76–82
 burns, 89–93
 cold sores, 86, 87
 dandruff, 83–86
 eczema, 88

psoriasis, 88
when to see the doctor, 86, 88, 91, 92
Sleep (see also Insomnia):
 and age, 163
 amount required, 161, 163
 quality of, 161, 163
Sleep-Aids:
 and alcohol, 166, 167, 168
 for children, 166
 drug of choice, 163, 164, 165, 166
 OTC ingredients, 164, 165, 166
 OTC not recommended, 169, 170
 OTC recommended, 168, 169
 side effects of, 164, 165, 167, 168
 warnings against, 164, 165, 166, 167, 168, 169, 170
Smoking:
 and cough, 23, 25, 26
 and eye irritation, 105, 107
 and indigestion, 35, 43
 and sore throat, 18
Sneezing:
 with allergies, 4
 with cold, 2
 with flu, 2
Soaps, abrasive, 79, 80
Soaps, acne, 80
Sore Throat (see also Throat):
 aspirin for, 19, 20
 causes of, 1, 2, 3
 in colds, 1, 2, 7, 12, 18, 19, 20
 cough drops, 18, 19, 21, 22
 diagnosis of, 19, 20
 fever and, 17, 19, 20
 gargling, 12, 18, 20
 hard candies, 18, 20
 lozenges, 18, 19, 21, 22
 from strep, 1, 3, 19, 20
 tonsillitis and, 3
 treatment, 7, 12, 17, 18, 19, 20
Speech, difficulty with, 119
Steam Inhalation, 12

Subject Index

Stomach:
  acidity, 37, 38, 42
  and aspirin, 42, 112, 113, 114, 116, 123, 128, 130, 135
  caffeine effects, 42, 43
  cancer, 37, 39
  cramping, 51
  diagram of, 36
  diseases of, 35
  "food rebound," 43
  gastritis, 35, 38, 39
  pepsin in, 39
Stomach Flu:
  symptoms, 50, 51
  viral cause, 50, 51
Stools:
  blood in, 37, 52, 59, 68, 69, 70
  loose, 46, 48–55
  mucus in, 50, 52, 59
  production of, 56
  tarry or black, 52, 59
Stool Softeners, 59, 60, 64, 65
  OTC products, 64, 65
Strep Throat:
  cause of, 1, 3, 19
  diagnosis of, 3, 19, 20
  duration of, 3
  fever and, 3, 19, 20
  symptoms, 3, 19, 20
  vs. tonsillitis, 3
  treatment for, 1, 20
Stroke, 58
Sun (see also Sunburn, Sunscreens, Sunshades):
  and acne, 79, 80
  diseases worsened by, 93
  drugs sensitive to, 93, 94
  and overexposure, 93, 105, 107, 110, 117
Sunburn (see also Burns):
  anesthetics for, 90, 94
  OTC not recommended, 95, 96
  OTC recommended, 94, 95, 96
  prevention of, 92, 93, 95, 96
  treatment of, 90, 91, 94, 95

Sunlamp:
  acne treatment, 79, 80
  burn treatment, 91
Sun Lotions:
  and sun lamps, 80
  and tanning, 92
Sun Poisoning (see Sun Sickness)
Sunscreens:
  correct use of, 92, 93
  effective ingredients, 92, 93, 95, 96
  how they work, 92
  OTC recommended, 92, 93, 95, 96
Sunshades:
  OTC recommended, 92, 97
  why they work, 92
Sun Sickness, 93
Swallowing Difficulty, 17, 37
  and bran, 61, 63

Tension:
  daytime sedatives for, 170, 171
  headache from, 110, 111, 112, 119
  and insomnia, 162
  premenstrual, 151, 152, 156, 157, 158, 159, 160
Throat (see also Sore Throat):
  mucous membranes of, 17, 18
  swallowing difficulty, 37, 61, 63
Thyroid Disease:
  aspirin and tests for, 116
  and cold remedies, 12, 15
  and constipation, 58
  and decongestants, 8
  and overweight, 142
Tonsillitis:
  cause of, 3
  duration of, 3
  other names for, 3
  vs. strep throat, 3
  symptoms of, 3
Trachoma, 104
Tranquilizers:
  and constipation, 58, 59

and sun sensitivity, 94
Traveler's Diarrhea, 51, 52
Tuberculosis, 25

Ulcers:
 aspirin and, 42, 116, 127
 eye, 104
 peptic, 37, 38, 39, 116
 self-treatment of, 39
 stomach, 35, 116
Upper Respiratory Infections (see Cold, common)
Urination:
 frequency of, 162
 and menstruation, 152
Urine, darkening of, 70
Uterus, 151, 153, 154
 relaxers for, 159, 160

Vasoconstrictors:
 in eye products, 106, 108
 in hemorrhoid preparations, 72, 73, 75
 side effects of, 72, 73
Veins:
 clots in, 69, 71
 in hemorrhoids, 67, 68, 69, 71
 varicose, 67, 139
 and vasoconstrictors, 72, 73
Virus:
 and antibiotics, 1, 18
 cold sores from, 20, 86–87, 93
 diseases caused by, 1, 2, 3, 9, 18, 19, 20, 25, 50, 51, 86, 104, 105
 herpes, 20, 86–87
 infectious mononucleosis, 20
 spreading, 7
 stomach flu, 50, 51
 trachoma, 104
Vision:
 blindness, 104
 double chill, 104, 118
 impairment of, 102, 104
 problems from sleep-aids, 164, 167
 serious symptoms of, 104, 118, 119
Vitamins:
 A and acne, 79
 absorption by mineral oil, 60
 B and alcoholism, 134
 B and anemia, 134
 C and colds, 5, 9, 10, 11
 in sedatives, 170
 side effects, 10, 11
 in sleep-aids, 165
 supplements, 149
Vomiting:
 from antihistamines, 168
 with blood, 37
 duration, 37
 with menstruation, 152
 with stomach flu, 50

Weight:
 chart of, 140
 diets to lose, 143, 144
 exercise effects, 142, 143
 gain with menstruation, 149, 151, 156, 157, 158
 loss with arthritis, 127, 128, 130
 loss as a serious symptom, 52, 60, 127, 128, 130
 maintenance of body, 141, 142, 143
White Head:
 cause of, 76, 78
 treatment of, 79

Yeasts:
 infections from, 20, 25
 monilia, 20

Drug Index

A and D Hemorrhoidal Suppositories, 72
A-Caine, 75
Acetaminophen, 20, 90, 112, 114, 115, 116, 122, 123, 130, 135, 136, 156
Acne, 76
Acne-Aid, 81
Acnederm, 81
Acne-Dome, 81
Acnesarb, 82
Acnomel, 80, 81
Adrinex, 149
A-Fil, 92, 97
Afrin, 8, 12, 13
Agoral, 61, 66
Albalon, 108
Alcohol, rubbing, 86
Alconefrin, 86
Alka-Seltzer, 41, 42, 47, 113, 120
Alka Seltzer Plus Cold Medicine, 14, 15
Alka-2, 46
Allerest Children's Tablets, 15
Allerest Eye Drops, 106, 108
Allerest Nasal Spray, 14
Allerest Tablets, 14, 15
Allerest Time Capsules, 14, 15
Allergesic, 14, 15
Alma Tar, 85
Aludrox, 40, 44
Aluminagel, 55
Aluminum Hydroxide, 54
Alva-Tranquil 8-Hour Timed Release, 164
Alva-Tranquil Regular, 164
Ambesol, 87
Amebil, 87
Americaine, 73, 75, 90, 91, 94

Amphetamines, 144, 145, 147, 149
Amphojel, 40, 46, 54
Anacin, 112, 120
Anahist, 15
Analbalm, 138
Analgebalm, 138
Anorexin, 149
Ansolysen, 59
Anti-B, 13
Anticoagulants, 116, 130
Antidepressants, 15
Antihistamines, 1, 9, 14
Anusol, 74
Apamide, 122
APC capsules, 121
APC tablets, 112, 117, 121
Appedrine, 149
Aqua-Ban, 150, 160
A.R.M. (Allergy Relief Medicine), 15
Arrestin, 33
Arthralgen, 123, 138
ASA capsules, 121
ASA tablets, 121
ASA Enseals, 121
Ascriptin, 120
Aspergum, 19, 121
Aspirin, buffered, 113, 120
Aspirin, plain, 7, 11, 12, 19, 20, 21, 30, 34, 42, 47, 90, 91, 112, 113, 114, 115, 116, 118, 119, 120, 121, 123, 127, 129, 130, 135, 136, 156, 164, 165, 171
Attapulgite, 55
Aureomycin, 94
Aveeno, 99, 100
Aventyl, 94
Axon, 14, 15

187

Drug Index

Axon Cough Medicine, 33
Axon Throat Lozenges, 22
Ayds, 146
Azo-Gantrisen, 94

Baby Oil, 96
Bacimycin, 95
Bayer Children's Cold Tablets, 15
Bayer Children's Cough Syrup, 32
Bayer Decongestant Tablets, 14
Bayer Non Aspirin Pain Reliever, 122
Bayer Timed Release Aspirin, 121
B.C. Powder, 120
B.C. Tablets, 120
Ben Gay, 138
Ben Gay Lotion, 138
Benoxyl, 80, 81
Benzedrine, 144
Benzocaine, 87, 90, 146, 147, 150
Benzophenone, 93, 96
Betadine Mouthwash/Gargle, 22
Betadine Shampoo, 84
Bio-Stik, 87
Bio-Tetra, 22
Birth control pills, 78, 156
Bisilad, 55
BiSoDol, 47
Blinx, 107
Blistaid, 87
Blister Klear, 87
Blistex, 87
Block Out, 93, 96
Bluboro, 99, 100
Brasivol, 80
Breck One Dandruff Shampoo, 85
Bromides, 163, 170
Bromo Quinine, 15
Bromo Quinine Cold Tablets, 15, 123
Bromo-Seltzer, 47, 117, 123
Bufferin, 113, 120, 128, 130
Burn-a-lay, 95

Burntame Spray, 94
Burrows Solution, 99, 100
Bur-veen, 99, 100
Butazolidin, 94

C-3, 16
Caffeine, 9, 120, 123
Caladryl, 101
Calamatum Spray, 101
Calamine lotion, 100
Calcium Carbonate and Soda, 47
Calm-Aids, 169
Calmol, 4, 74
Calotabs, 65
Camalox liquid, tablet, 44
Campho-Phenique, 87
Camphor, 137
Cankaid, 87
Capron, 121
Carter's Little Pills, 65
Cascara, 62
Castor Oil, 61, 66
Cenac, 81
Cenagesic, 15, 16
Cepacol, 22
Cepacol Lozenges, 21
Cepacol Troches, 22
Cheracol D, 31
Chinoform, 52
Chloraseptic, 21, 22
Chlor-Trimeton Decongestant, 15
Chlor-Trimeton Expectorant, 32, 33
Citrocarbonate, 47
Clean 'N Treat, 95
Clearasil, 81
Clearasil Regular Tinted, 81
Clearasil Vanishing Formula, 81
Clear Eyes, 106, 108
Clopane Hydrochloride Solution, 13
Clove oil, 137
Clyserol, 62, 63
Clyserol Oil Retention Enema, 62, 66
Cocoa Butter, 72, 96

Drug Index

Coconut Oil, 96
Codeine, 59, 156
Codimal DM, 32, 33
Colace, 60, 64, 70, 74
Coldene Children's Cough Formula, 32, 34
Coldene Adult's Cough Formula, 33, 34
Colgate 100, 22
Collyrium, 107
Coloctyl, 64
Colrex, 15, 16
Colrex Syrup, 32, 34
Colrex Troches, 22
Comfortine Ointment, 100
Compazine, 94
Compoz, 169
Conar, 32
Conar-A Suspension, 32, 34
Conar Expectorant, 32
Congespirin, 121
Contac, 15, 16
Contac Jr., 16
Contac Nasal Mist, 8, 14
Contique Artificial Tears, 108
Contrablem, 81
Cope, 121
Coricidin, 15
Coricidin Cough Formula, 32, 34
Coricidin 'D', 7, 9, 15, 16
Coricidin Demilets, 15, 16
Coricidin Medilets, 15
Coricidin Nasal Mist, 8
Correctol, 64
Cortisone, 91, 99
Coryban-D, 13, 15, 33, 34
Cosadein, 33
CoTylenol, 7, 15, 16
Covangesic, 16
Counterirritants, 137, 138
Creamalin, 41, 44
Creo-Terpin, 33
Creo-Terpin Plus, 33
CZO Lotion, 100

Dalicote, 101
Dalidyne, 87
Dandricide Shampoo, 84
Danthron, 62
Datril, 122, 136
Decadron, 116
Declomycin, 94
Decongestants, 7, 8, 9, 11, 13
Deep Strength, 138
Degest, 106, 108
Delcid, 44
Demazín, 16
Denorex Shampoo, 85
Devarest, 169
Dexatrim, 150
Dexedrine, 144
Dextromethorphan, 28, 31
Dexule, 147, 150
Diabinese, 94, 116
Dialose, 64
Dicarbosil, 46
Dicumerol, 116
Diet-Trim, 147, 150
Di-Gel, 41, 42, 44
Dilantin, 94
Dimacol, 33
Diocte (DSS) 64
Dio Medicone, 64
Diothane, 75
Disonate, 65
Diuretics, 94, 147, 150
Diurex Day-Span Water Capsules, 150
Diurex Water Pills, 147
Diuril, 94
Dr. Caldwell's Senna Laxative, 62, 65
Domeboro, 99, 100
Dondril Anticough Tablets, 33
Donnagel, 55
Donnagel-PG, 55
Dorana, 75
Dorcol Pediatric Cough Syrup, 33
Dormin, 169
Double Danderine, 84
Doxan, 62
Doxinate, 60, 65
Drest, 84
Dristan, 7, 9, 15
Dristan Cough Formula, 33, 34
Dristan Nasal Mist, 14

Drug Index

Dristan Tablets, 16
Dristan Time Capsules, 15, 16
Dri-Toxen, 101
Dry and Clear W/N–12, 81
Duadacin, 16
Ducon, 44
Dulcolax, 62, 65
Dulcolax Suppository, 62, 66
Duration, 8, 12

Effersyllium, 53, 55, 61, 63, 64
Empirin Compound, 112, 117, 121
Enden Shampoo, 85
Endotussin-C, 34
Endotussin-NN, 34
Eno, 41, 47
Enteroquinol, 52
Enterovioform, 52
Epsom Salts, 61
Esidrix, 94
Espotabs, 65
Eudicane, 73, 75
Excedrin, 112, 123
Excedrin, P.M., 121, 123
Ex-Lax, 61, 65
Exocaine, 138
Exocaine Plus, 138
Extendac, 15, 16
Eye Cool, 108
Eyegenic Eye Mist/Drops, 108
Eye Stream, 107

Fedrazil, 16
Feen-A-Mint, 61, 65
Femcaps Capsules, 160
Fendon, 122
Figure Aid, 150
Fizrin, 41, 42, 47, 120
Flavihist, 15, 16
Fleet, 62, 63, 65, 66
Fleet Enema Oil Retention, 62, 63, 66
Fletcher's Castoria, 65
Fomac Cream Cleanser, 85
Fostex, 81
Fostex Cake Bar, 85
Fostril, 80, 81
4Way Cold Tablet, 7, 16, 121
4Way Nasal Spray, 14
Fulvicin, 94

Gantrisin, 94
Gaviscon, 47
Gelumina, 44
Gelusil, 41, 44, 128, 130
Gelusil-M, 44
Gentlax, 62
Gluco-Fedrin, 13
Glycerin Suppositories, 62, 66
Glyceryl Guaiacolate, 28, 31
Grapefruit Diet Plan Tablets, 150
Griseofulvin, 94
G-W Emulsoil, 61, 66

Haley's M-O, 61, 66
Head & Shoulders, 85
Heet, 138
Hemor-Rid Rectal Ointment, 75
Histadyl EC, 34
Histavite-D Cough Syrup, 33, 34
Hungrex, 147, 150
Hydrocil, 61, 63, 64

Ice-O-Derm, 82
Inversine, 59
Iodo-Enterol, 52
Ionax, 82
Ionil, 85
Ionil T, 85
I-Sedrin Plain, 13
Isodettes (junior, plain, super), 22
Isodine Mouthwash/Gargle Concentrate, 22
Isophrin, 12, 13
Isopto Alkaline, 108
Isopto-Frin, 108
Isopto Plain, 108
Isopto Tears, 109
Ivarest, 101

Jergens Clear Complexion Gel, 82

Drug Index

Johnson & Johnson First Aid Cream, 94

Kalpec, 52
Kao-Con, 52
Kaolin, 52, 53, 54, 55
Kaolin-Pectin with Paregoric, 55
Kaolin-Pectin, suspension, 52, 53, 54
Kaoparin with Paregoric, 53, 55
Kaopectate, 52, 53, 54
Kaopectolin, 54, 55
Kaopectalin with Paregoric, 55
Kip First Aid Spray, 95
Kip Hemorrhoid Relief, 73, 75
Kip Moisturizing Lotion, 95
Kip Sunburn Spray, 90, 94
Klaron, 81
Klaron Lotion, 85
Kolantyl, liquid, tablet, wafer, 44
Komed Mild, 82
Kondremul, 66
Konsyl, 61, 63, 146

Lacril, 109
Lanacane Creme, 73, 75
Lavoris, 22
Liquifilm Tears, 109
Liquimat, 81
Listerine, 22
Listerine Cough Control, 22
Listerine Throat Lozenges, 21
Loroxide, 81
Lotioblanc, 82
Lyteers, 109

Maalox (suspension), 41, 44, 45, 128, 130
Maalox No. 1, 45
Maalox No. 2, 45
Maalox Plus, 42, 45
Magnesium-Aluminum Hydroxide Gel (USP), 41, 47
Malcogel, 45
Mazon Shampoo, 85
Measurin, 121
Medicane Dressing Cream, 95
Medicated Face Conditioner (MFC), 82
Menthol, 137
Mentholatum Deep Heating Lotion, 138
Mentholatum Deep Heating Rub, 138
Metamucil, 53, 54, 55, 61, 63, 64, 70, 74, 146
Meted Shampoo, 85
Meted 2 Shampoo, 85
Methyl Salicylate, 137
Metrecal, 145
Mexaformo, 52
Micrin Plus, 22
Midol, 121, 160
Midran Decongestant, 15, 16
Miles Nervine, 170
Milk of magnesia, 59, 61, 63
Milk of magnesia-mineral oil emulsion, 66
Mineral oil, 60, 66, 96
Minit-Rub, 138
Mistol, 16
Mistol with Ephedrine, 13
Mistol Mist, 14
Monique Dandruff Control Shampoo and Rinse, 84
Mucilose, 53, 55, 61, 63, 64
Murine, 108
Murine 2, 106, 108
Mylanta, 41, 42, 44, 45
Mylanta II, 41, 45
Myotrain, 95

Naldetuss, 33, 34
Naphazoline, 106
Naphcon, 106, 108
Nasal Sprays, 8, 12, 13, 14
Naso Mist, 14
Nature's Remedy, 62, 65
Nebs, 122, 135, 136
NegGram, 94
Neo-Cultol, 66
Neoloid, 61, 66
Neo-Synephrine, 8, 12, 13, 14
Neo-Synephrine Compound, 15, 16
Neo-Synephrine Elixir, 16

Drug Index

Nervine Effervescent, 170
Nioform, 52
Nite Rest, 164, 169
Nopramin, 94
Nose Drops, 8, 12, 13, 14
Novafed, 16
Novafed A, 16
Novahistine with APC, 7, 9, 15, 16
Novahistine Elixir, Fortis, or Melet, 15, 16
Novahistine Expectorant and DH, 33, 34
Noxzema Skin Cream, 80, 82, 94
Noxzema Sunburn Spray, 95
NTZ, 14
Nujol, 66
Nupercainal, 73, 75
NyQuil, 33, 34
Nytol, 164, 169

Ocusol, 105, 106
Ocusol Drops, 108
Ogilvie Anti-Dandruff Shampoo, 84
Olive oil, 96
Op-Isophrin, 108
Orinase, 94, 116
Ornacol, 16
Ornex, 16
Oxy-5, 80, 81
Oxymetazoline, 8

Pabafilm, 93, 96
Pabagel, 95
PABA-TAN, 96
PAC, 121
Panalgesic, 138
Pan-Oxyl-5, 81
Para-aminobenzoic acid (PABA), 92, 93, 96, 97
Parafilm, 96
Paregoric, 53
Parepectolin, 53, 55
Pargel, 54
Parke-Davis Throat Discs, 21
Pazo, 75
Pectin, 52

Pektamalt, 54
Penetro Cough and Cold Medicine, 33, 34
Penicillin, 20
Pepto-Bismol, 41, 47
Percodan, 59
Perifoam, 75
Pernathene, 150
Pernox, 80
Persadox, 81
Pertofrane, 94
Pertussin 8 Hour Cough Formula, 33
Pertussin Plus Night-Time Cold Medicine, 33, 34
Petrogalar, 66
Petro-Syllum No. 1 & No. 2, 66
Phenacetin, 117, 121, 160
Phenergan, 94
Phenol, 87
Phenolax, 61, 62, 65
Phenolphthalein, 61
Phenylephrine, 7, 8, 106, 108
Phillips Milk of Magnesia, 40, 46, 61, 65
pHisoAc, 81
pHisoDan, 85
pHisoderm Medicated Liquid, 82
Phosphal-jel, 41
Phospho-Soda, 63, 65
piSec, 81
Plova, 55, 64
PNS, 75
Poison Ivy Cream, 101
Polymagma, 55
Pontocaine, 95, 101
Pondosan, 147, 150
Post 40%, 61, 63
Post Raisin Bran, 61, 63
Pragmatar, 86
Prednisone, 116
Prefrin, 108
Preludin, 162
Pre-Mens Forte, 159, 160
Preparation H, 72, 75
PreSun, 92, 96
Privine, 14
Pro-Banthine, 59

Drug Index

Pro-Blem, 82
Prolamine, 150
Pronac, 82
Proval, 122
Proval drops, 122
Psorex, 86
Psychic energizers, 16, 162
Psyllium, 53

Quartets, 15, 16
Queltuss Tablets, 31
Quiet World, 169

Rectalgan, 75
Rectal Medicone, 75
Reducets, 147, 150
Regulin, 61, 63, 64
Regutol, 65
Relax-U-Caps, 169
Reserpine, 94
Resinol, 94
Resorcinol, 80
Resorcitate, 85
Resulin, 81
Rezamid, 82
Rezamid Shampoo, 85
Rhuli, 101
Rhulihist, 101
Rinse Away Shampoo, 84
Robitussin-CF, 33
Robitussin Cough Calmers, 32
Robitussin Cough Tablets, 32
Robitussin-DM, 32
Robitussin-PE, 33
Rolaids, 40, 41, 47, 159
Romex, 33
Romilar, 16
Romilar Capsules, 33, 34
Romilar CF, 34
Romilar Children's Cough Syrup, 32
Romilar III, 33
Romotin, 52

St. Joseph Aspirin, 120
St. Joseph Children Decongestant, 16
St. Joseph Cold Tablets for Children, 16
St. Joseph Fever Reducer for Children, drops & elixir, 122
Sal Hepatica, 61, 63, 65
Salicylamide, 120, 123, 164
Salicylic Acid (see also Aspirin), 80
San-Man, 164, 169
Scadan, 84
Scopolamine, 163, 164, 169, 170
Sea & Ski, 93, 96
Sebacide, 82
Sebacide Lotion, 82
Sebaveen, 85
Sebulex, 85
Sebutone, 86
Sedacaps, 169
Seedate, 169
Sego, 145
Selenium Blue, 85
Selenium Sulfide, 85
Selsun Blue, 85
Senna, 62
Senokot, 62, 65, 66
Seret, 84
Serpasil, 94
Serutan, 61, 63, 64
Shark Liver Oil, 72
Silain-Gel, 45
Silence is Golden, 32
Simethicone, 42, 45
Sinarest, 15, 16
Sine-Aid, 121
Sine-Off, 13, 15, 16, 121
Sinuseze, 16
Sinustat, 15, 16
Sinutab, 9, 15, 16
Sinutab II, 16
SK-APAP, 122, 135
Sleep-Aid, 169
Sleep-Eze, 169
Sleepinal, 169
Slender, 145
Slender-X, 147, 150
Slim-Mint, 146, 150
Sloan's Liniment, 138
Slumberette, 169
Snootie, 96

Drug Index

Soda Mint, 47
Sodium Bicarbonate, 41, 47, 159
Solarcaine, 95
Solarcaine Lip Balm, 87
Solar Cream, 92, 97
Solbar, 93, 96
Soltice, 14
Sominex, 164, 169
Sominex 2, 169
Somnicaps, 169
Soothe, 108
Sorbutuss, 32
Sparine, 94
SPD Analgesic Cream, 138
SPD Liquid, 138
Spec-T, 22
Spectrocin, 95
Squibb Milk of Magnesia, 46, 65
S.T. 37, 22
Stanback Powder, 120
Stanback Tablets, 120
Stanco, 120
Stelazine, 94
Stri-Dex Medicated Pads, 82
Sucrets, 21
Sucrets Cold Decongestant, 16
Sucrets Cough Control, 22
Sudafed Syrup, 16
Sulfur, 80, 81
Sulfur-8 Conditioner, 85
Sulfur-8 Shampoo, 84
Sunril, 160
Super Anahist, 9, 15, 16
Super Anahist Nasal Spray, 14
Supercitin Sugar-Free Cough Syrup, 34
Super Shade Lotion by Coppertone, 96
Sure-Sleep, 169
Sure Tan, 96
Surfak, 60, 65
Syllamalt, 55, 64

Tackle, 82
Tame Creme Rinse, 84
Tanac, 87
Tear-efrin, 108
Tearisol, 109
Teenac, 82
Tega-Caine Aerosol, 90, 94
Tegretol, 94
Tegrin Shampoo, 86
Tempra, 112, 114, 115, 122, 130
Tempra drops, 122
Tenuate, 162
Terramycin, 94
Tetrahydrozoline, 106
Therapads Plus, 82
Thorazine, 59, 94
Thylox PDC, 84
Thymol, 137
Ting, 82
Titanium dioxide, 92
Titralac, 40, 47, 159
Toclonol Expectorant, 32
Tofranil, 59, 94
Top Brass Cream, 84
Tranquilizers, 166, 168, 170, 171
Tranquim, 169
Tranquinol, 170
Travad, 62, 66
Trendar, 160
Triaminic Expectorant, 33, 34
Triaminicin Tablet, 14, 15, 16
Triaminic Syrup, 15, 16
Tricreamalate, 47
Tridione, 94
Trigesic, 123
Trilafon, 94
Trilium, 122
Trind, 33, 34
Trind-DM, 33, 34
Trisogel, 47
Trisol Eye Wash, 107
Trokettes, 22
Tuck's cream, ointment, 75
Tuck's Saf-Tip, 66
Tums, 40, 41, 46
Tussagesic Suspension, 33, 34
Tussagesic Tablets, 33, 34
Tylenol, 12, 20, 90, 112, 114, 115, 130, 136, 156
Tylenol drops, 122
Tylenol Extra Strength, 122

Drug Index

Ultra Tears, 109
Unguentine Ointment "Original Formula", 94, 95
Unguentine Plus, 95
Unguentine Spray, 95
Uval Sun 'n' Wind Stick, 96
Uval Sunscreen Lotion, 93, 96

Vacuetts, 66
Valadol, 122
Valgesic, 122
Vanoxide, 81
Vanquish, 112, 123
Vanseb, 85
Vanseb-T Tar, 86
Vaseline Hemorr-Aid, 75
Vaseline Carbolated Petroleum Jelly, 95
Vaseline Pure Petroleum Jelly, 70, 72, 91, 95
Vasominic TD, 16
Vicks Day Care, 16
Vicks Formula 44 Cough Mixture, 33
Vicks Formula 44-D, 33
Vicks Inhaler, 14
Vicks NyQuil Nighttime Colds Medicine, 16
Vicks Sinex, 14
Vicks Sinex Long Acting Decongestant Spray, 8, 12, 13
Vicks Vapo Steam, 27, 31
Vicks Va-Tro-Nol, 14
Vioform, 52
Visine, 106, 107, 108
Vitamin A, 79
Vitamin C, 5, 9, 10, 11

Warfarin, 116
Wey-Dex, 147, 150
Willard's Tablets, 47
Wingel liquid, tablet, 45
Wyanoids Suppositories, 72, 75

X-11 Reducing Agents, 150
Xerac, 82

Zepheran, 105
Zetar, 86
Zincon, 84
Zinc Oxide, 92, 97
ZP-11, 84
Ziradryl, 101

About the Author

A graduate of Columbia University's College of Physicians & Surgeons, Dr. Rubinstein, a neurologist, is presently Associate Clinical Professor of Neurology at U.C.L.A. in California.